FIRST PLACE BIBLE STUDY

PRESSING ON to the PRIZE

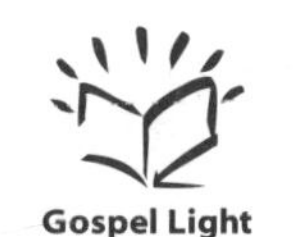

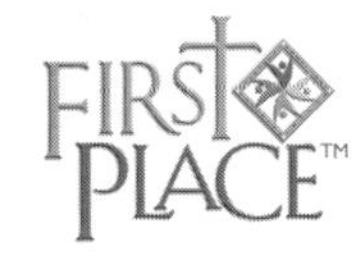

Gospel Light is an evangelical Christian publisher dedicated to serving the local church. We believe God's vision for Gospel Light is to provide church leaders with biblical, user-friendly materials that will help them evangelize, disciple and minister to children, youth and families.

It is our prayer that this Gospel Light resource will help you discover biblical truth for your own life and help you minister to others. May God richly bless you.

For a free catalog of resources from Gospel Light, please contact your Christian supplier or contact us at 1-800-4-GOSPEL *or* www.gospellight.com.

PUBLISHING STAFF
William T. Greig, Chairman
Kyle Duncan, Publisher
Dr. Elmer L. Towns, Senior Consulting Publisher
Pam Weston, Senior Editor
Patti Pennington Virtue, Associate Editor
Jeff Kempton, Editorial Assistant
Hilary Young, Editorial Assistant
Bayard Taylor, M.Div., Senior Editor, Biblical and Theological Issues
Barbara LeVan Fisher, Packaging Concept and Design
Samantha A. Hsu, Cover and Internal Designer

ISBN 0-8307-2926-7

Printed in the U.S.A.

CAUTION

The information contained in this book is intended to be solely informational and educational. It is assumed that the First Place participant will consult a medical or health professional before beginning this or any other weight-loss or physical fitness program.

CONTENTS

FOREWORD

My introduction to Bible study came when I joined First Place in March of 1981. I had been in church since I was a small child, but the extent of my study of the Bible had been reading my Sunday School quarterly on Saturday night. On Sunday morning, I would listen to my Sunday School teacher as she taught God's Word to me. During the worship service, I would listen to our pastor as he taught God's Word to me. Digging out the truths of the Bible for myself had frankly never entered my mind.

Perhaps you are right where I was back in 1981. If so, you are in for a blessing you never dreamed possible. As you start studying the truths of the Bible for yourself, you will see God begin to open your understanding of His Word. Bible study is one of the nine commitments of the First Place program. The First Place Bible studies are designed to be done on a daily basis. Each day's study will take approximately 15 to 20 minutes to complete, but you will be discovering the deep truths of God's Word as you work through each week's study.

There are many in-depth Bible studies on the market. The First Place Bible studies are not designed for the purpose of in-depth study. They are designed to be used in conjunction with the other eight commitments of the program to bring balance into our lives. Our desire is for each member to begin having a personal quiet time with God each day. This time alone with God should include a time of prayer, Bible reading and Bible study. Having a quiet time is a daily discipline that will bring the rich rewards of balance, something we all need.

A part of each week's study is the Bible memory verse for the week. You will find a CD at the back of this Bible study that contains all 10 of the memory verses for the study set to music. The CD has an upbeat tempo suitable for use when exercising. The songs help you to easily memorize the verses and retain them for future reference. If you memorize Scripture as you study, God will use His Word to transform your life.

Almost every First Place member I have talked with about the program says, "The weight loss is wonderful, but the most important thing I have received from my association with First Place is learning to study God's Word."

God bless you as you begin this exciting journey toward a balanced life. God will richly bless your efforts to give Him first place in your life. Remember Matthew 6:33: "But seek first his kingdom and his righteousness, and all these things will be given to you as well."

Carole Lewis
First Place National Director

INTRODUCTION

The First Place Bible studies were developed to be used in conjunction with the First Place weight-loss program. However, the studies could also be used by anyone who desires to learn more about God's Word and His will, with the added bonus of learning more about living a healthy lifestyle.

A Balanced Life

First Place is a Christ-centered health program, emphasizing balance in the physical, mental, emotional and spiritual areas of life. The First Place program is meant to be a daily process. As we learn to keep Christ first in our lives, we will find that He is the One who satisfies our hunger and our every need.

God's Word contains guidelines for maintaining our physical well-being, equipping us mentally to make right choices, providing emotional stability to handle everyday circumstances as well as crisis situation, and growing spiritually as we deepen our relationship with Him.

The Nine Commitments

The First Place program has nine commitments that will help you draw closer to the Lord and aid you in establishing a solid, consistent and healthy Christian life. Each commitment is a necessary and important part of the goal of First Place: to help you become healthier and stronger in all areas of your life and live the abundant life He has planned for you. To help you achieve growth in all four areas, First Place asks you to keep these nine commitments:

1. Attendance
2. Encouragement
3. Prayer
4. Bible reading
5. Scripture memory verse
6. Bible study
7. Live-It plan
8. Commitment Record
9. Exercise

The Components

There are six distinct components to this Bible study to aid you in bringing balance to your life. These components include the 10-week Bible study, 6 Wellness Worksheets, 2 weeks of menu plans, the leader's discussion guide, 13 Commitment Records and the Scripture memory CD.

The Bible Study

Each week of each 10-week Bible study is divided into five daily assignments with days 6 and 7 set aside for reflections on the week's lesson. The following guidelines will help make your study more enjoyable and profitable:

- Set aside 15 to 20 minutes each day to complete the daily assignment. It's best not to attempt to complete a week's worth of Bible study in one day.
- Pray before each day's study and ask God to give you understanding and a teachable heart.
- Keep in mind that the ultimate goal of Bible study is not for knowledge only but also for application and a changed life.
- First Place suggests using the *New International Version* of the Bible to complete the studies.
- Don't feel anxious if you can't seem to find the *correct* answer. Many times the Word will speak differently to different people, depending upon where they are in their walk with God and the season of life they are experiencing.
- Be prepared to discuss with your fellow First Place members what you learned that week through your study.

Wellness Worksheets

The informative and interactive Wellness Worksheets have been developed by Dr. Jody Wilkinson of the Cooper Institute in Dallas, Texas. These worksheets are intended to help you understand and achieve balance in all four areas of your life: physical, mental, emotional and spiritual. Your leader will assign specific worksheets as At-Home Assignments throughout the 13-week session.

Menu Plans

The two-week menu plans were developed especially for First Place by Chef Scott Wilson. Each menu is meant to simplify meal planning and include food exchanges. These meals are based on the MasterCook software that uses a database of over 6,000 food items, which was prepared using United States Department of Agriculture (USDA) publications and information from food manufacturers.

Leader's Discussion Guide

This discussion guide is provided to help the First Place leader guide a group through this Bible study. It provides information for the leader to prepare for each weekly group meeting.

Personal Weight Record

The Personal Weight Record is for the member to use to keep a record of weight loss. After the weigh-in at each week's meeting, the member will record any loss or gain on the chart.

Commitment Records

Thirteen Commitment Records (CRs) are provided in the back of this Bible study. For your convenience these have been printed on perforated paper so that you may easily remove them from the book and carry them with you through each week as you keep your First Place commitments. Directions for filling out the CRs precedes those pages.

Scripture Memory Music CD

Since Scripture memory is such a vital part of the First Place program, the Scripture memory CD for this study is included in the back inside cover. The verses for this study are set to music that can be listened to as you work, play or travel. The CD can be an effective tool as you exercise since the first verse is set to music with a warm-up tempo, the next eight verses are set to workout tempo, and the music of the last verse can be used for a cooldown.

FORGETTING THE PAST

Week One

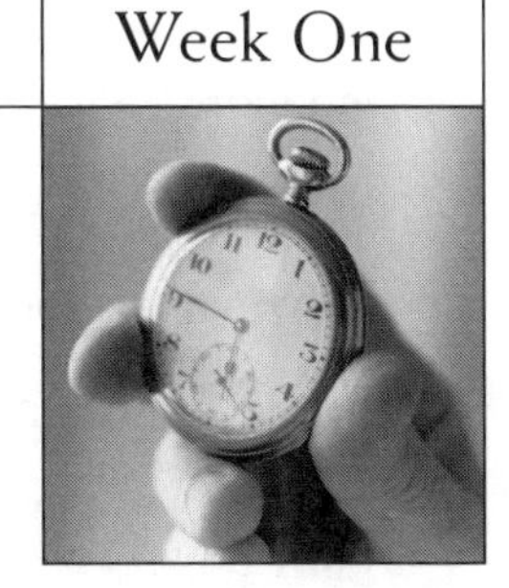

MEMORY VERSE

I press on toward the goal to win the prize for which God has called me heavenward in Christ Jesus.

Philippians 3:14

Today is the first day of your journey toward the future. Your goal is the prize for which God called you. Philippians 3:13 sets the stage for this journey. "But one thing I do: Forgetting what is behind and straining toward what is ahead."

This Bible study will show you how to leave behind past failures and conditions. With God's help, you will press on toward the future, keep your commitments and attain the prize God keeps for you.

DAY 1: *Gaining Freedom from What Holds You Back*

What holds you back from gaining the prize? When you joined First Place, you made a commitment. Prayer, Bible study and memorizing God's Word will guide you toward the prize. Revelations 21:5 (*NKJV*) says, "Behold, I make all things new."

Whether this is your first or eighth session, it is a new beginning. Forget what has happened in the past. Focus on the newness of this journey. Cast off your yoke of slavery to the past. Galatians 5:1 states, "It is for freedom that Christ has set us free. Stand firm, then, and do not let yourselves be burdened again by a yoke of slavery." Don't let the burdens you carry from the past keep you from moving forward.

Focus on the future, new events and new relationships by forgetting what may have held you back in the past. God does.

- Underline the key words in the following phrase from Jeremiah 31:34 that express what God promises to forget about you:

  "For I will forgive their wickedness and will remember their sins no more."

- Do your sins cause God pain?

  ☑ Yes ☐ No

- How do you feel when someone sins against you and causes you pain?

  heartbroken, grief

If you are hurt by another's actions against you, how much more is God hurt when we sin against Him? Yet He forgives us and remembers the sin no more.

- According to Ephesians 4:32, how are we to forgive one another?

  Just as God forgave us

- In light of God's forgiveness of you in Christ, is there anyone you need to forgive? Write the person(s) name or initials here.

  Amy, my mother

If God has forgiven you, then you must forgive those who have hurt you. Ask yourself if you have truly forgiven the person.

- What can you do to insure this forgiveness? Of the following, check all that apply:

  ☐ Seek counseling.
  ☐ Make a phone call.
  ☐ Write a letter.
  ☐ Go to the offender.
  ☑ Pray about it.
  ☑ Make changes in my life.
  ☑ Spend time in God's Word.

If you have not truly forgiven that person and let go of the hurt, do it this week. Then you will forge ahead with God's abiding presence in you.

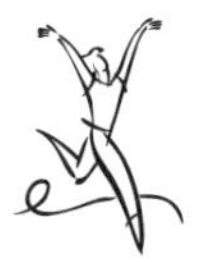

Thank You, Father God, for forgiving me and loving me when You sent Your Son.

Thank You, God, for this opportunity to begin anew.

Commit to learning your memory verse this week by listening to the CD and repeating the verse as you exercise, drive or go about your daily activities. Keep your eyes on the prize.

DAY 2: *Avoiding the Temptation of Looking Back*

Now that you are on the journey, be careful not to give in to the temptation of looking back. Read Luke 9:62. These words of Jesus remind us to keep our minds off past failures and focus on Him.

You may have negative events in your own life. If you dwell on them, they become like sores that fester. If instead you use what you learned from the experience and how God brought you through it, you can enrich the lives of others who may have the same struggle.

- What are some negative events in the past that you find yourself looking back on even today?

embarrassing times.
sins of adolescents

When Jesus called His disciples in Matthew 4:18-22, they left their business-as-usual lives to follow Him. God calls you to follow Him.

- Where were you at the time you first heard God's call?

Church revival

- What did you hear God saying to you?

tugging at my heart to walk
c Him.

➳ How long did it take you to respond?

A day or possibly two

➳ Who and/or what did you leave behind?

Looked ahead Awareness of living for God now.

➳ What must you leave behind to follow the commitments of First Place?

Bad habits.

Our joy comes in knowing when to use the past and when to forget it, answer His call and follow Him. Genesis 19:15-26 tells about a person who did not resist the temptation of looking back.

➳ How did Lot's wife disobey God?

By looking back

➳ What were the consequences of looking back?

death

➳ Is it just as offensive to God for us to look back with thoughts such as *if only, I should have* or *why didn't I*?

☐ Yes ☐ No

➳ Why or why not?

We need to learn but not dwell on past mistakes.

What are the possible consequences if you continue to look back? Check those that apply.

- ☐ Depression
- ☐ Frustration
- ☐ Bitterness
- ☐ Resentment.
- ☐ Anger
- ☐ Envy
- ☐ Regret
- ☐ Grief
- ☐ Jealousy
- ☐ Longing

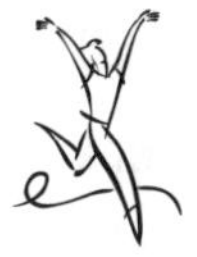

Lord, keep me from dwelling on negative past events and give me a genuine reconciliation with the past because I know You can make all things new.

God, help me use past experiences in a positive way to encourage others.

DAY 3: *Breaking Free from the Grips of Others*

If you are allowing God to be in control, then others cannot cause you to fail. Some people in your life might want to see you fail in controlling your habits rather than see you succeed. Others may control your time in such a way that you neglect exercise, prayer and Bible study. Some may place temptation in your way. When your commitments to First Place are not fulfilled, you sense failure. See how Joseph was faced with temptation in Genesis 39:1-20.

How did Joseph respond to the temptation of Potiphar's wife?

Refused

What or who keeps you from controlling your health and dietary problems? Describe the situation.

Me + my craving for junk food in the afternoon or ~~food~~ for too much food in the evening.

- What in your life is controlling you by tempting you away from prayer and Bible study?

fatigue, T.V.

- What circumstances or events keep you from exercising?

Time + fatigue

In Matthew 15:17-20, Jesus tells us that what comes out of our mouths has much more impact than what goes into our mouths. Encouraging words to others keep you from being an obstacle for them in reaching their goals.

Even as Joseph had a clear perception as to God's purpose at work in his life, even so must you see God's plan for your life. Let Him be in control of all situations and temptations. Don't give in to circumstances or events, but rely fully on Him. Use your recovery from past failures or negative circumstances to tell others how they, too, can let God be in control.

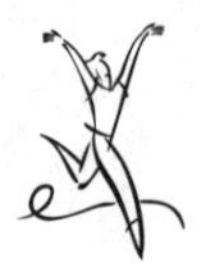

Father God, I seek Your help in giving me strength to face temptation.

Lord, develop the strengths You have begun in me and reveal other areas of strength I need to develop.

DAY 4: *Picking Up After Life's Shipwrecks*

God is able to accomplish good in our lives, even when it seems that things in life are not fair! Paul had committed his whole life to serving Christ. He was seeking a just trial as a Roman citizen when he and those with whom he was traveling were shipwrecked. Read the story of their experience in Acts 27:13-44.

- What dangerous situation did Paul and those traveling with him face?

death

➳ How did Paul find hope in this situation (see vv. 21-25)?

thru prayer

Paul believed God would fulfill His purpose even though the circumstances of shipwreck seemed to say otherwise. As a way of forgetting the past, you too can focus on the new life God gives as you pick up the pieces after a tragedy. The positive action is much healthier than the negative reactions of blaming and grieving over life's losses.

➳ Think of a time in your life when you felt shipwrecked emotionally. What did you experience?

sadness, hopelessness, grief, despair, loss

➳ What was the outcome?

➳ What helped you get through the emotional shipwreck?

➳ Have you allowed your health to become poor? How are you going to pick up the pieces of this situation and go forward?

Read Acts 27:44. Note how God accomplishes His purpose in our lives even through difficult experiences if we trust Him.

➳ How can you use your experience to witness to others about God's grace and love?

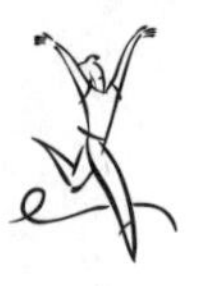

Lord God, help me to deal with the unresolved problems of my life.

Father, when my life is a shipwreck, give me Your guidance.

DAY 5: *Remembering to RSVP to God's Invitation*

Jesus offers us an invitation to new life in Him. All are invited, but not all respond when the invitation is extended. Read John 8:1-11. The crowd pointed their fingers of condemnation at the woman. Compared to the woman, people in the crowd felt smug. After Jesus confronted them, they must have felt very small. Jesus opened the door to a new life for the woman.

- Notice the Lord's invitation to the woman in John 8:11. What was His command to her?

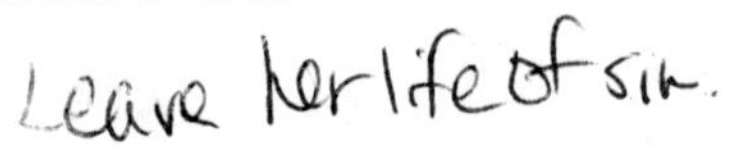

- Rank the following reasons from 1 to 4 (with 1 being the most likely) in order of the most likely excuses someone might use for not responding to Jesus' invitation for a new life:

___ Too good to be true	___ Too painful to let go
___ Too bad to be forgiven	___ Too mad to give up offenses

Read 2 Samuel 9:1-13. Mephibosheth was afraid to meet King David because his grandfather Saul had opposed David being named king and had even tried to kill David.

- What was Mephibosheth's handicap?

Crippled

- What was David's reason for returning Saul's land to Mephibosheth and inviting Mephibosheth to eat at the king's table from now on?

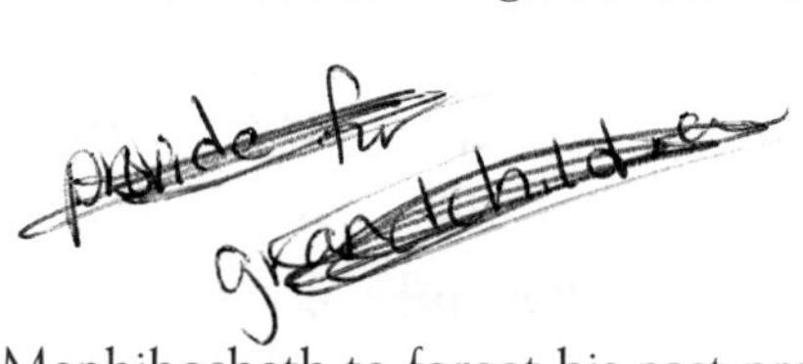

- Why did David want Mephibosheth to forget his past problems?

Very few people have a past as bad as Mephibosheth's. It seemed that he would never be able to get away from the fact that he was crippled and that his grandfather had tried to kill David. He must have been terrified to accept the king's summons. Have you turned down God's invitation to new life because you were afraid of your past? Look at the blessing that Mephibosheth almost missed.

Many things in the past need to be forgotten. We can choose to refocus our attention and energies on better things. God is always faithful to show us His footprints in every season of our lives.

The story of Mephibosheth illustrates the inestimable grace of God. The following paraphrase of 2 Samuel 9:7 conveys a message from the heart of God to help you overcome your pains from the past: "Don't be afraid, for I will surely show you kindness for the sake of my Son, Jesus."

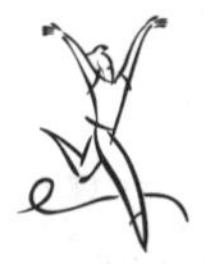

Thank You, God, for Your great mercy to me.

Thank You, God, for the good things, people and events in my past. Renew my spirit and dedication to use whatever You want from my past for whatever You want to do in my future.

Day 6: *Reflections*

Romans 3:23 tells us that every one of us has sinned. No one sinner is any worse than any other in God's eyes. He invites all to join Him for the feast in heaven. When you accept Him, verse 24 is His gift of grace, for you are "justified freely by his grace through the redemption that came by Christ Jesus."

If this is your first session with First Place, you will learn to use the Scriptures as you pray. Beth Moore's book *Praying God's Word* teaches us how to pray in this way.[1] If you are in a repeat session, utilize what you have already learned about praying the Scriptures.

Since God so freely forgives you through Jesus Christ and forgets your sins and remembers them no more (see Hebrews 8:12), you must forgive yourself for past failures. Beth Moore tells us that when you let past sins and failures of any kind become a stronghold, it "sets itself up against the knowledge of God."[2] She says, "A stronghold is anything that exalts itself in our minds, pretending to be bigger or more powerful than our God."[3] The stronghold may be an addiction, an unforgiving spirit toward a person who has hurt you, despair over a loss or anything that consumes so much of your emotional and mental energy that your abundant life is strangled.

- Which areas of the commitments have given you a problem in the past because of strongholds in your life? Check those that apply.

  - ☐ Prayer
  - ☐ Bible study
  - ☐ Memorizing Scripture
  - ☐ Scripture reading
  - ☐ Live-It plan
  - ☑ Exercise
  - ☐ Encouraging others
  - ☐ Commitment Record
  - ☐ Attendance

Choose one commitment to concentrate on for next week. While working on all of them, add one new one each week for particular attention and prayer. When you pray, keep Scriptures in mind. Beth Moore tells us that prayer and the Word are our two primary sticks of dynamite. Strapping them together and igniting them with faith in what God says He can do will help you overcome any stronghold on your life.[4]

The key to freedom from strongholds is in 2 Corinthians 10:3-5. Read this passage carefully. You can "demolish arguments and every pretension that sets itself up against the knowledge of God, and . . . take captive every thought to make it obedient to Christ" (v. 5). Using the divine weapons God has given you, pray using God's Word. The following are examples of Scripture prayers you can use today:

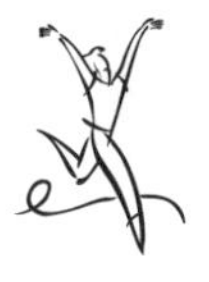

Father God, help me to forget my past failures and press on to the prize for which You have called me heavenward. Help me to focus on pressing forward with You now (see Philippians 3:14).

Lord, help me to use Your Word as a weapon against the temptations of the flesh because Your Word is quick and powerful and sharper than any two-edged sword. Your Word pierces me even to my soul. Your Word is a discerner of the thoughts and intents of my heart (see Hebrews 4:12).

Day 7: *Reflections*

This week's study has focused on the aches, pains, miseries and failures of the past. You have been encouraged to go forward in the process of leaving the past behind. When Jesus calls and you answer by following Him, He will show you the blessings that come from obedience.

When you share past experiences where God helped you to overcome tragedy or unwelcome circumstances, you show forth God's glory, and He will lead you into new fields and give you new adventures.

Another thought from Beth Moore is that you "can take your thoughts captive, making them obedient to Christ, every time you choose to think Christ's thoughts about any situation or stronghold instead of Satan's or your own."[5] She says that praying the Scriptures will give you an intimate communication with God. Let your mind be retrained or renewed and think His thoughts about your situation rather than your own.

Focus on the prayer of each promise He gives you in the Bible.

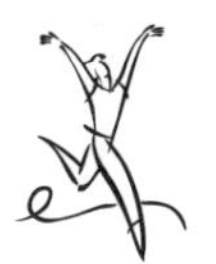

Thank You, Father, for not giving me a spirit of timidity, but a spirit of power, of love and of self-discipline (see 2 Timothy 1:7).

Help me, Father, to trust You when I am tempted because You promised that no temptation has seized me except what is common to man. And You are faithful and You will not let me be tempted beyond what I can bear. But when I am tempted, You will also provide a way out so that I can stand up under it (see 1 Corinthians 10:13).

Heavenly Father, I press on toward the goal to win the prize for which You have called me heavenward in Christ Jesus (see Philippians 3:14).

Notes

1. Beth Moore, *Praying God's Word* (Nashville, TN: Broadman and Holman, 2000).
2. Ibid., p. 3.
3. Ibid.
4. Ibid., p. 6.
5. Ibid., p. 7.

GROUP PRAYER REQUESTS TODAY'S DATE:______________

NAME	REQUEST	RESULTS

STRAINING TOWARD THE FUTURE

Week Two

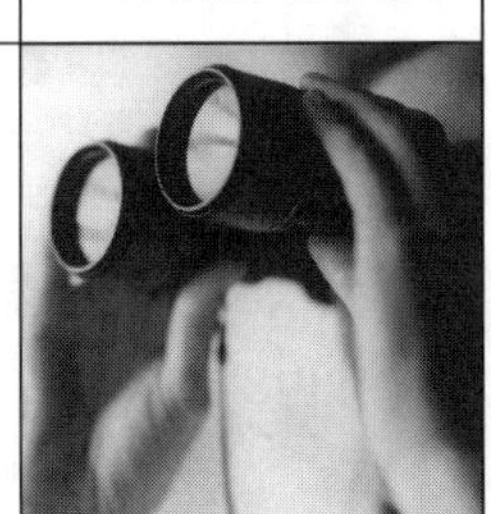

MEMORY VERSE

By faith Abraham, when called to a place he would later receive as an inheritance, obeyed and went, even though he did not know where he was going.

Hebrews 11:8

As you work toward your First Place goals, this week's memory verse encourages you to follow in the footsteps of faithful Abraham. He obeyed when called and went even though he didn't know specifically where he was going. He forgot his past and pressed on into the future for a place whose architect and builder was God (see Hebrews 11:10).

Lean forward to the life God is building for you. With Him as your leader, you will succeed.

DAY 1: *A Place That Is Not Known*

A visit to our nation's capital, Washington, D.C., can bring about a surge of patriotism and renewed commitment to responsible citizenship.

In a similar manner, Hebrews 11 serves as a shrine to the Christian faith. You read about the great heroes of faith and their relationship to God. God called Abraham, and his response was to follow obediently into the unknown. God calls you to a future He has planned for you. He is leading you on a journey with a heavenly destination.

- According to Hebrews 11:8, what did Abraham have to do in order to possess his inheritance from God?

obeyed and went

- What do you need to do in order to receive your inheritance from God?

obey and follow

You, like Abraham, must have faith and be willing to obey God.

- Do you have the faith that God will help you reach the health and spiritual goals you have set for yourself in First Place?

☑ Yes ☐ No

- According to Hebrews 11:10, who was the architect and builder of the place which Abraham was looking forward to receiving?

God

- What is the inheritance toward which you are traveling in obedience to God?

?

God is the planner and builder of your inheritance. Your part is to believe His promise and obey His call. The details of the future may be unknown to you, but you can be assured that God is in control.

- In Jeremiah 18:1-6, God showed the prophet Jeremiah how He lovingly and firmly shapes the lives of his children. Number the following events from this passage in chronological order.

2 Jeremiah watched the potter work at his wheel.
1 God told Jeremiah that He would give him His message.
4 God said that His people were like clay in His hand.
3 The potter shaped the pots as it seemed best to him.

➳ Briefly describe some evidence in your life right now that God is shaping you and molding you and holding your future securely in His hands.

selling our house

Consider 1 Peter 1:3-9, which says that you have an inheritance "that can never perish, spoil or fade—kept in heaven for you."

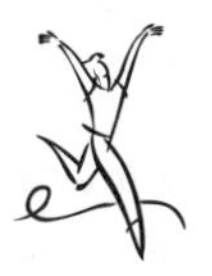

God, You know my fears about my future. Help me to overcome fear of the unknown.

God, make me more pliable in Your hands.

DAY 2: *A Destination to Be Shown*

In Genesis 12:1-9, you will find the original account of Abraham (Abram) following God's call. This story describes how Abraham kept on his journey by his faith in God's direction. Hebrews 11:8 points out that Abraham had such confidence in God's selection that he "obeyed and went"—evidently without hesitation.

➳ Based on Genesis 12, number the following events in chronological order:

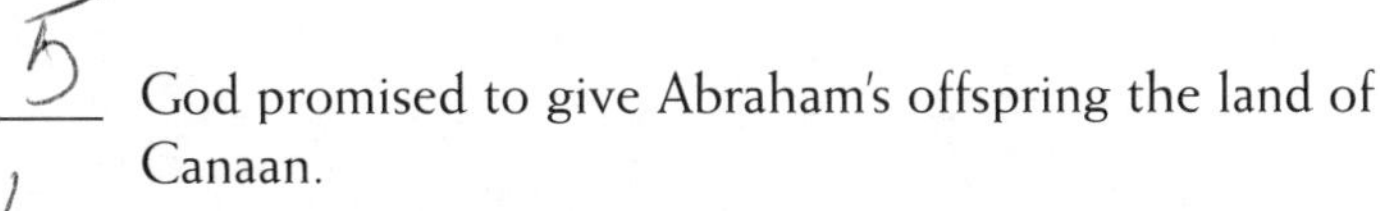

__5__ God promised to give Abraham's offspring the land of Canaan.
__6__ Abraham built an altar to God at Bethel.
__3__ Abraham left Haran as God commanded.
__1__ God commanded Abraham to leave his father's household.
__4__ Abraham set out for the land of Canaan.
__2__ God promised to make Abraham a great nation.

Genesis 12:4 records one of the most interesting facts about Abraham's journey.

- How old was Abraham when he set out from Haran in obedience to God?

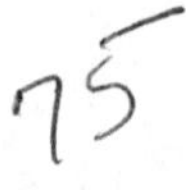

- Why do you think we are told how old he was?

Show how settled he was

- As a vessel being molded by God, how resistant are you toward what He wants you to be? Circle the answer that best applies to you.

some none a lot a little

- If God has not already revealed His plan for your life, do you feel it's because He probably doesn't have any definite plans for you? Explain.

- What does Jeremiah 29:11 tell you about God's plan for your future?

Plans to prosper us

- How does Abraham's story and God's promise in Jeremiah give you greater confidence that God will reveal His future plans for you in a timely manner?

He says He will

Abraham's faith was not a shot in the dark, but a step into the light!

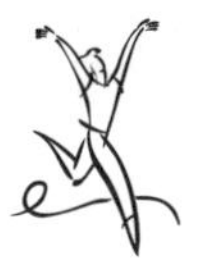

God, help me have confidence in You and Your plans for me.

God, give me the willingness to obey Your call to follow Your plans for my future.

DAY 3: *A Home That Is Not Your Own*

When a husband is transferred to another city or country because of his job, the wife usually follows with their family. They become strangers in another place. Hebrews 11:9 makes a pointed statement about Abraham's home: "By faith he made his home in the promised land like a stranger in a foreign country." If Abraham felt like an outsider, imagine how Sarah must have felt.

- Circle some of the feelings you think Sarah might have had about this journey.

excited	confused	uncertain	doubtful
fearful	exhilarated	isolated	

- How do these feelings match some of your own on your journey?

- Do any of the commitments you made to First Place—such as exercise, cutting back on portion size, daily Bible study and memorization of Scripture—seem too difficult because you are not accustomed to doing them?

Even though Hebrews 11:11-12 describes Abraham and Sarah as "past age" and "barren," God promised them a future worth striving for. It's never too late to trust God. Sarah learned to trust God to keep His promises.

- What caused Sarah to believe that God would keep His word?

- What did God do for Abraham and Sarah that was humanly impossible?

Whatever fears Sarah or Abraham might have had, obeying God was their priority. Have you expected positive experiences along your spiritual journey? A significant step forward in personal faith occurs when trusting God surpasses needing to feel good about faith decisions. Although Abraham felt like a stranger in a foreign land, his new home was in the Promised Land. Read the memory verse (Hebrews 11:8) again but also include verse 9.

- Match the following Scriptures that remind us that obedient actions often lead to difficult circumstances:

____	Luke 9:58	a. Our faith is tested by fire to purge impurities.
____	John 15:19	b. Jesus Himself had no place to lay His head.
____	Isaiah 1:25	c. The world hates Christians as it hated Jesus.

- Are you surprised when difficulties and trials result from your obedience to God? Explain.

In *My Utmost for His Highest*, Oswald Chambers wrote, "The one passion of Paul's life was to proclaim the Gospel of God. He welcomed heart-breaks, disillusionments, tribulation, for one reason only, because these things kept him in unmoved devotion to the Gospel of God."[1]

What is your passion? Good food? Nice clothes? A good job? A nice home? Any passion other than one for God will cause you to stumble and falter in your journey. Don't be surprised by setbacks and disappointments, but remember that you never face these difficulties alone. God is always with you.

In 2 Corinthians 5:7, Paul warned us to "live by faith, not by sight." Abraham demonstrated walking by faith and not by sight. He obediently set forth on the journey God planned for him.

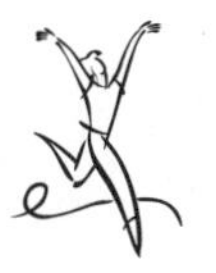

God, help me to walk in Your light. Guide my path.

God, help me to accept disappointments and setbacks as a reminder to always trust in You and Your plans for my life.

DAY 4: *A Promise from God's Holy Throne*

Hebrews 11:10 specifies the motivation that gave direction to Abraham's adventure: "He was looking forward to the city with foundations, whose architect and builder is God."

Just as Abraham, you don't have the blueprints for your own future, God does.

Reread Jeremiah 29:11. God knows what He has planned for your life. All He asks is that you put every area of your life in His loving hands for all your future needs. Many other Old Testament men and women followed God's plan for their lives. Esther, Joseph, Moses, Samuel are a few who listened to God, obeyed and were leaders of their people. One woman in particular in the Old Testament learned to trust God for her future when her present was in shambles. Two caring people, Naomi and Boaz, assisted her in discovering God's plans for her life.

The book of Ruth tells the story of Naomi, a woman who had lost her husband and sons, one of whom was married to Ruth. These two widowed women set out on a journey to a new home. In Ruth 3:3-6, Naomi gave Ruth some advice.

➳ How did Ruth respond to the advice Naomi gave her?

➳ How can that attitude help you realize the plan God has for your life?

Obey without question and be blessed.

God's promise for the future kept Abraham going.

➳ What was God's promise to Abraham in Genesis 12:2-3?

To bless him.

Since Abraham had no children at the time, Abraham's faith journey is even more significant. Even before the births of his son Isaac and his grandsons Jacob and Esau, Abraham had faith in God's promise. He knew that God had promised him a great nation, but without children it seemed that the nation couldn't come from him. But the heavenly Father had a plan that even Abraham and Sarah considered impossible. God was faithful to fulfill His promises to them (see Genesis 21:1-2).

➳ According to Isaiah 6:8, what was Isaiah's answer when he heard God's call?

Send me

The vision God gave the apostle John in Revelation 5:11-14 energized John with an exalted view of God personally at work in his life.

Just like Isaiah and John, Abraham was called to action in his journey with God.

➳ Are you sensing that God has a specific purpose for your life? What is it?

Yes, ?

➳ What are some actions you need to take to respond to His purpose for you?

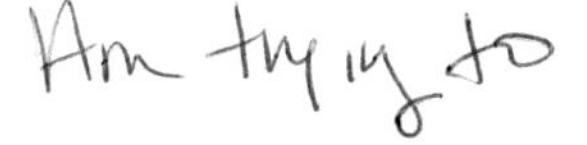

A children's minister assembled a support group for children. All seven members of the group had lost a parent by death or divorce. At the last group session, this minister gave a plaque to each child. On it was written Jeremiah 29:11, with each child's own name in place of the word "you."

➳ Make this verse more personal for you by writing it here and putting your name in place of "you."

Claim this verse as God's personal promise to you. In Revelation 3:20, He asks to come into your life. Have you accepted His invitation to let Him be Lord of your life? If so, thank Him for including you. If not, consider letting Him reign in your life beginning today.

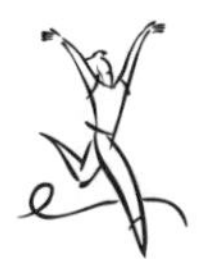

Lord, come into my life in a new and wonderful way.

God, I claim Your promise for my life. Guide me on my journey with You.

DAY 5: *A City That Surely Stands*

When Abraham obeyed God's call, he may not have known where he was going, but he knew what he was looking for. Hebrews 11:10 says, "For he was looking forward to the city with foundations, whose architect and builder is God." Abraham knew that he had an eternal future with his God. As you continue this week's study on straining toward the future, keep your attention focused on the eternal city—your final destination.

- What is a destination or goal that you have set for yourself?

Since Abraham lived only in tents, he was drawn into the future by his attraction to a spectacular city. God calls you to the destinations of healthful, faithful and useful living. If you are content to stay where you are, you will not reach your destination. If you follow His call, God will give you the foundation of His truth and presence on which to build.

- What do you need to do in order to reach your goal?

probably more

Jeremiah 29:11 was initially given to the people of Israel, who were in desperate need of an encouraging word from God. Read the whole context in Jeremiah 29:1-14.

- Why did the Israelites need these promises from God and what did He promise them?

- How can these promises help you in your current situation?

- According to Matthew 6:19-21, why should you not "store up for yourself treasures on earth"?

- Why do you need to "store up for yourselves treasures in heaven"?

When we store treasure in heaven, we demonstrate our commitment to a lifestyle that is pleasing to Him and the eternal city that awaits. The saying "Rome wasn't built in a day" reminds us that most things worth having take a considerable amount of time to complete. This maxim applies to your spiritual life as well. God patiently works out His plan for your eternity.

- How can you demonstrate your commitment to reach the goal God has for you through First Place?

In your prayer time today, make a list in your journal of those things for which you can be thankful to God. List people, events and/or things.

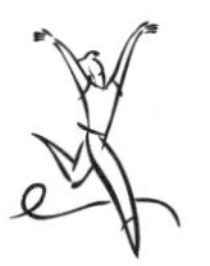

God, thank You for the strength You give me to reach the destination You have for me.

God, thank You for Your love and guidance in every area of my life, including my First Place commitments.

DAY 6: *Reflections*

During the past week you read about men and women who put their complete trust in God to lead them with loving hands. They are examples of what God can do in the lives of those who obey and follow him. God builds your future with loving hands, just as He did for those of the Old Testament.

- Read through the First Place commitments. Which one(s) has God helped you with this week in a special way or a new way? Check all that apply.

☐ Prayer
☐ Bible study
☐ Memorizing Scripture
☐ Scripture reading
☐ Attendance
☐ Exercise
☐ Encouraging others
☐ Commitment Record
☐ Live-It plan

God used Boaz and Naomi to help Ruth discover His plan for her life. They were a positive influence.

➳ Who are some people God has used in your life as a positive influence?

➳ How did they influence you?

Are there people you know who need a word of encouragement or support? Make a special effort to write a note of encouragement to each one, telling how you are thinking about and praying for him or her.

Pray the following Scriptures to give you courage in witnessing to others:

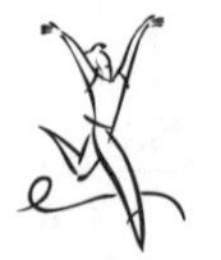

Help me Lord, to share Your Word and not to be ashamed of the gospel of Christ, for I know it is the power of God for the salvation of everyone who believes (see Romans 1:16).

Lord, take over my speech and my witness. Let me speak words not of human wisdom, but let them be a demonstration of the Spirit's power so that my faith is not resting in the wisdom of men, but in Your power, Almighty Father (see 1 Cointhians 2:4-5).

Father God, help me in my witness to others. Forbid my boasting in anything except in the cross of my Lord Jesus Christ, by whom the world has been crucified to me, and I to the world (see Galatians 6:14).

DAY 7: *Reflections*

This week's study has focused on how God uses people and events in our lives to help us find the way in our journey toward the prize that God has for us through Christ Jesus. He has shown us how he supplies all our needs through His Son, Christ Jesus. Paul knew this without a doubt.

Consider Philippians 4:19. God is the source from which all your needs can be filled. He also promised in Psalm 37:4 that if you delight in Him, He will give you the "desires of your heart."

He knows your needs before you ask and promises that if you seek Him, you shall find Him; ask and it will be given, knock and it will be opened to you (see Matthew 7:7).

Seek God through His Word. Commit His words to memory and call them to mind when you need to make any supplication to Him. Whether you need help to break down a stronghold, strength to meet temptation or guidance to solve a problem, God is faithful to His Word. With His Word sealed in your heart as your very own, you equip yourself with weapons that Satan cannot face. He will flee in fear when he hears you pray using God's Word.

Seek God's wisdom and guidance in His promises as you pray these Scriptures.

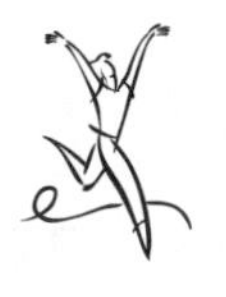

Father God, I know You are my God for ever and ever; You will be my guide even to the end (see Psalm 48:14).

Lord, help me to acknowledge You in all my ways so that You might direct my path (see Proverbs 3:6).

Almighty Father, help me to be continually with You so that You will hold me by my right hand. You will guide me with your counsel, and afterward receive me to glory just as You promised (see Psalm 73:23-24).

Lord, instruct me and teach me in the way I should go. I know You will counsel me and watch over me (see Psalm 32:8).

Lord God, give me the faith of Abraham who was willing to go where You called him for his inheritance, even though he didn't know where he was going (see Hebrews 11:8).

Note

1. Oswald Chambers, *My Utmost for His Highest* (Grand Rapids, MI: Discovery House, 1994), n.p.

Group Prayer Requests Today's Date:______________

Name	Request	Results

PRESSING ON IN THE PRESENT

Week Three

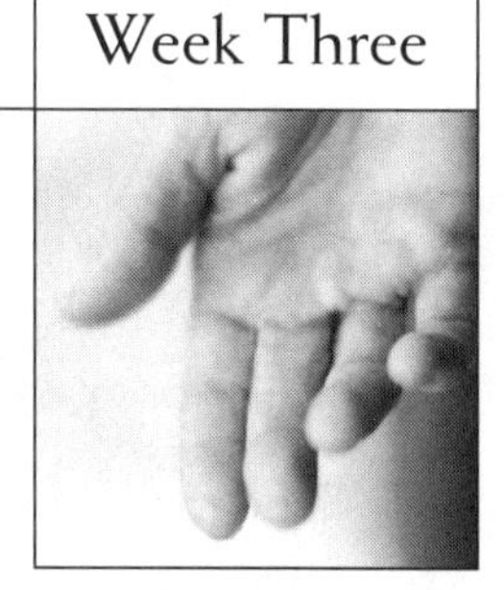

MEMORY VERSE

But the worries of this life, the deceitfulness of wealth and the desires for other things come in and choke the word, making it unfruitful.

Mark 4:19

In this study so far, you have dealt with two major areas of pressing on to the prize. The first week you learned to forget the past and then last week to press toward the future. These two life skills are essential in moving toward the goal you wish to reach.

In this week's study, you will discover the heart of the matter by pressing on in the present. The past is past, the future unknowable, but the present is now and it is your focus.

DAY 1: *Asking for What You Need*

Pressing on in the present begins with asking for what you need for today. James instructs believers to ask God for provision.

➳ According to James 1:5-7, what can you ask God to provide?

Wisdom

➳ How does God give wisdom when we ask?

➳ Considering James 4:1-3, what are some reasons believers might hesitate to ask God for their needs?

Both our failure to ask and asking with the wrong motives block God's blessing in our lives. God cares about every aspect of your life. You can ask your Father for exactly what you need.

➳ Write the promise found in Philippians 4:13 in your own words.

➳ In Mark 10:46-52, Bartimaeus dared to ask Jesus for exactly what he needed from Him. Mark the following events as T (for true) or F (for false):

____ Jesus asked him what he wanted.
____ Bartimaeus was standing by the side of the road.
____ Others encouraged him to call out to Jesus.
____ He told Jesus he wanted to see.
____ He reluctantly came to Jesus.
____ He followed Jesus after receiving his sight.

Bartimaeus clearly asked Jesus for what he needed.

➳ Write what you need most right now for spiritual victory.

This week strive to review the memory verse regularly. Use the *Walking in the Word* book and the CD to cement this week's verse in your mind.

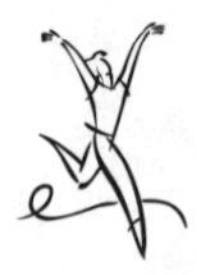

Father, help me pray not for my own desires but with a heart that believes You shall supply all my needs through my riches in Jesus Christ.

DAY 2: *Throwing Away Excuses*

Excuses provide barriers that keep you from attaining the goal you set. They get in the way so that you don't press on, and they sap your strength. Used long enough, the barrier may become a stronghold in your life. A stronghold is anything that keeps you from doing the things God wants you to do for successful living in the present. The excuses put make-believe limitations on what you think you can achieve.

Read John 5:1-15. Here you find a handicapped man who had an excuse for not going in to the pool for healing. When Jesus offered him an opportunity for healing, he used the excuse, "I have no one to help me." Perhaps he was using this problem as an excuse for not making needed changes in his life.

- What excuses are you using for your eating problems?

I deserve this.

- Have you experienced a time in your life when you felt that you had no one to help you? How did God help you in that time?

yes. Sent me help. Made me lean on Him.

Notice that Jesus didn't focus on what had happened to the man in the past or the fact that he had no one to help him. Above all things, Jesus wanted to know, "Do you want to get well?" The paralyzed man didn't realize that his answer to Jesus' question was more powerful than any of his own limitations. Jesus, in effect, was saying that what you want is more important than what is holding you back. You can take a positive step, and miracles will happen. "Get up! Pick up your mat and walk."

- Look back at the excuses you listed above. What needs to happen in order for you to give up your excuses?

Another barrier preventing you from accomplishing your goals may be the destructive comments from others that often deter your progress in pressing on in the present. If you find yourself in this predicament, take heart. You are not alone.

In 1 Samuel 17:26-33, David's older brother Eliab accused David of being conceited, irresponsible and wicked. Even King Saul joined in discouraging David.

- What did Saul say about David's chances of defeating Goliath?

You are not able

David had to overcome these negative comments in order to follow God's leading. Read Matthew 5:11. Christians are often laughed at or scorned because of their beliefs. These negative comments and reactions can hurt and discourage. Standing firm in your beliefs will bring the blessings God promised.

- Has there been a time in your life when you were falsely accused or a time when you were scorned or belittled because of your beliefs? Briefly describe it.

- How did God help you in this situation?

God will give you the patience and strength you need to endure such suffering.

- What does Peter tell us about suffering in 1 Peter 2:19-21?

Is good if it is for God

➳ Why is it more commendable to suffer for doing good? God says So. May be should suffer for doing wrong.

You will continue pressing on in the present when you patiently endure false accusations, ridicule or scorn, or when you habitually throw away excuses. Just as the testimony of the invalid changed from not having anyone to help him to a confession that Jesus made him well, your excuses will fall away, and your detractors will disappear when you confess to Jesus that you need His help. Realize that you can't keep your commitments alone. God will help you.

At the same time, be careful that you are not a barrier to someone else. Let your words be encouraging to others who may be having difficulty. Call a fellow First Place member and encourage him or her on his or her journey.

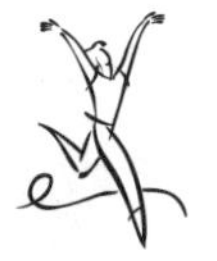

Lord, help me to stop the excuses and focus on You. Let me be a testimony of faith in what You can do in my life.

DAY 3: *Overcoming Obstacles Along the Way*

Even as you grow in your ability to get rid of habitual excuses and throw off destructive comments, other obstacles may appear along the way. Both internal and external roadblocks can hinder your progress in pressing on in the present. By God's grace and in God's strength, you can gloriously overcome these seemingly insurmountable obstacles. Your obstacles become God's opportunity to do something wonderful and enriching in your life. The decisions you make in the light of your roadblocks clarify how committed you are to pressing on.

In Mark 2:1-12, the paralytic man in Capernaum had external problems to overcome in order to get to Jesus. Jesus healed him because the man had help from his friends to overcome the crowds around Jesus.

➳ How did God use the man's friends to help him get to Jesus?

they took him to Jesus

Check the external obstacles that are weights to your spirit.

- [ ] Financial burdens
- [x] Health concerns
- [x] Time pressures
- [ ] Aging parents
- [x] Child care
- [ ] Other ____________

The four men who carried the paralytic man to Jesus displayed compassion, commitment, cooperation and creativity.

How have friends helped you in a difficult situation and brought you closer to God?

Which of the character qualities—compassion, commitment, cooperation or creativity—do you feel is strongest in you?

Compassion

Which quality do you need the most from others?

You must put forth persistent effort toward your obstacles just as this man's friends were persistent in their efforts to get the paralytic to Jesus. Before he could be fully healed, Jesus addressed the internal obstacle that kept the man from being healed completely—his sin (see Mark 2:5,9-12). This message is important: God is concerned about your spiritual needs as well as your physical ones. In First Place you can renew the inward person as well as the outward appearance.

What internal needs serve as obstacles to your spiritual growth? Check any that apply.

- [ ] Resentment
- [ ] Anger
- [x] Rebellion
- [ ] Unforgiving spirit
- [x] Unwilling spirit
- [ ] Lack of faith

How does God want to help you deal with those needs?

↑ self discipline

Remember that the deepest sin can't rise above the love that was expressed at Calvary. Christ died for you and forgives you when you seek Him and ask Him to remove the obstacles keeping you from pressing on in the present. Our loving heavenly Father is attentive to our every need. Nothing is impossible to God.

Review the memory verse for this week. Say it aloud to yourself or to a friend. Pray that the obstacles listed will not come in and choke the Word for you.

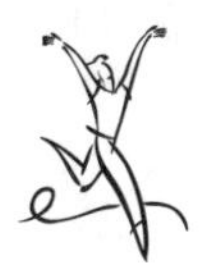

Heavenly Father, help me to prevent the worries of my life, the deceitfulness of wealth and the desire for other things from coming in and choking out Your Word and making me unfruitful.

God, help me to overcome the obstacles in my life, so I can have victory and press on to the prize You have for me through Your Son, Jesus.

DAY 4: *Finding Armor That Fits*

Paul delivered a very strong challenge for pressing on in the present when he encouraged the believers at Ephesus.

- How does Ephesians 6:10-11 clarify what is required to have God's strength and power in daily living?

full armor of God

Ephesians 6:10-18 tells us how to equip and arm ourselves to stand against the schemes of the devil. The moment-by-moment victorious Christian life requires the adept use of each part of God's armor to combat Satan's maneuvers.

- Read Ephesians 6:10-18. Match the physical piece of armor to its corresponding Christian quality.

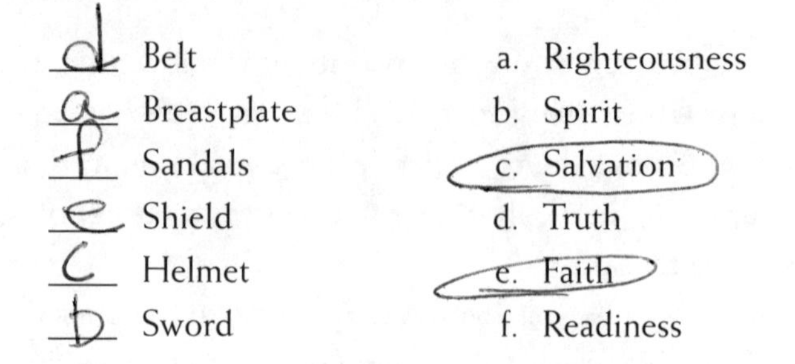

d	Belt	a.	Righteousness
a	Breastplate	b.	Spirit
f	Sandals	c.	Salvation
e	Shield	d.	Truth
c	Helmet	e.	Faith
b	Sword	f.	Readiness

- Using the same list, circle the qualities that you feel God has developed in your life to this point; then give an example of how God has used one of them in your life.

Although prayer is not listed as a separate piece of armor, it is given the encompassing power to cover all the rest. The full armor of God prepares the believer to stand firm when evil attacks. Prayer provides mental and spiritual alertness on all occasions to not be caught off guard.

- In verse 18, what does Paul say about prayer?

pray continuously about everything

- Now give attention to any spiritual quality you were not able to circle. Boldly tell God which piece of armor you would like to put on.

Spirit of His word.

- What steps are you willing to take to see that this happens?

Study

- How can these spiritual weapons help you to overcome your poor eating or exercise habits?

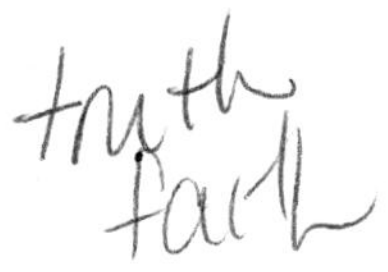

Today's lesson challenges you to put on the full armor of God. Your Commander in Chief offers armor that fits you completely. Suit up and stand firm!

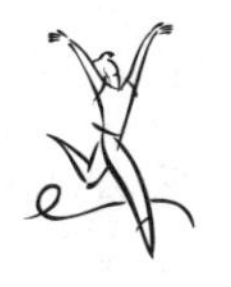

Lord, help me stand firm in the armor You have supplied for me to fight my battles.

Lord, help me pray with all power and supplication in the Spirit that I may open my mouth boldly to tell others of You.

DAY 5: *Fighting the Giants*

In Numbers 13:17-33, when the Israelite spies considered the strength of their enemies, they felt very small, like grasshoppers among giants.

- What did the spies tell the Israelites about the Promised Land?

- Which two men believed they could conquer the land? What were their reasons?

- Why were the people of God so easily defeated by the enemies of God?

The story of David and Goliath is a familiar one to most people. The decision you make to let God lead you into battle is directly in proportion to how you are pressing on in the present.

In 1 Samuel 17:8-11, David found himself among grasshoppers in the presence of a giant named Goliath. There wasn't one giant slayer in the whole army until David came along! David refused to give in to fear as Saul's army, who were terrified and dismayed, had done. Instead, he stood up with faith as a giant slayer.

David had confidence in the weapon he possessed.

- Read 1 Samuel 17:45. What was David's weapon?

- What situation has asserted itself as a giant to mock you and defy the power of God in your life?

- What do you think is necessary to transform you from a grasshopper into a giant slayer?

Sometimes bad circumstances occur, and you are knocked down. Paul and Barnabas experienced an emotional roller coaster on their first missionary journey to Lystra. Read Acts 14:8-23. Paul went from being hailed as a god in verses 11 and 12 to being attacked by a hailstorm of stones thrown at him in verse 19. Courage caused him to get up and go back into the city. Commitment to God's kingdom caused him to return to Lystra.

- What actions of Paul can be an encouragement to believers to pick themselves up when life's circumstances knock them down (vv. 19-23)?

➳ Which of those actions have helped you get up when you have been knocked down?

In Acts 16:1-5, on his second missionary journey, Paul returned to Lystra where he had been stoned and left for dead. There he discovered Timothy. Timothy soon became Paul's son in the faith. Had Paul not been able to pick himself up when he had been knocked down, he may have never returned to Lystra and found this special person.

➳ In your own words, write Paul's glowing testimony in Philippians 2:19-23 about the discipleship of Timothy.

Believes in the interest of Jesus Christ

Call or write to encourage someone in your First Place group today. A phone call or card of encouragement is important in helping to pick up someone when they are down.

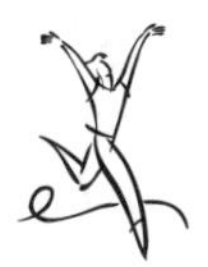

Lord, give me the courage to go on, to pick up the pieces, and to trust in Your name when I am faced with giants and adversity in life.

Dear Lord, may the words of my mouth be a testimony of Your power and grace in my life.

Day 6: *Reflections*

During this week's study you read about men who faced adversity and obstacles in serving God. They called on His name, remained faithful and found victory.

You have two weapons to fight the battles against the giants that rise up against you. Those weapons are prayer and God's Word. You learned about using His Word in prayer to help you overcome the external as well as internal handicaps that keep you from reaching your goal.

What if the paralyzed man's friends had given up because the crowd was too big to get into the house where Jesus was? What a blessing would have been missed. The same is true of the Israelites. If they had listened to Joshua and Caleb, they would have moved into the Promised Land 40 years sooner. Don't listen to those who criticize you and want you to fail. They will keep you from reaching your goal. Have courage and call upon the name of the Lord to overcome your foe.

As you pray today, use the following Scriptures as examples:

Lord, help me to be strong and wait on You, for I know You will strengthen my heart (see Psalm 27:14).

Heavenly Father, though I stumble, I will not fall, for I know You uphold me with Your hand (see Psalm 37:24).

Lord, You are my rock, my fortress and my deliverer. You, God, are my strength, in whom I will trust; my shield and the horn of my salvation, and my stronghold (see Psalm 18:2).

DAY 7: *Reflections*

This week's study has focused on how God uses obstacles and setbacks to help you learn to press on. The computer is one of the most timesaving inventions in history. If you want to get to a program quickly, it offers shortcuts so you don't have to go through a menu and wait. You have a shortcut to God when you are knocked down by life's challenges and feel worry or fear. That shortcut is praising God in prayer. When you are busy praising God for the things you have, what you don't have decreases in importance. Praise in Scripture and prayer will open you up to God's presence—your shortcut to peace.

Memorizing God's Word has a value that is immeasurable. Look at how Jesus Himself faced temptation. Read Matthew 4:1-11. How powerful the Word of God is when battling Satan. He cannot stand and fight when faced with Scripture.

Memorizing Scripture will help you handle difficult situations, overcome temptation and give you guidance. When you pray through Scripture, you personalize the verse by putting your name in key places and translating it into your own words. This will give you ownership over the verse.

No one can be effective if he or she tries to break down a stronghold with carnal weapons such as determination, secular psychology or denial. These may work for short periods, but the strongholds won't fall. Strongholds must be demolished, destroyed. What is it that is keeping you from focusing on God and makes you feel overpowered? Anything that consumes so much of your emotional and mental energy strangles your abundant life. Isn't this Satan's ultimate goal?

Use the following Scripture prayers as examples of how to break down the strongholds in your life:

Lord, let me boldly speak out and say that You, Lord, are my helper, and I will not fear what man shall do to me (see Hebrews 13:6).

Oh, Lord, You are my God; I will exalt You and praise Your name, for You have done wonderful things for me. Thank You for loving me (see Isaiah 25:1).

Father, help me to accept my momentary troubles because they are achieving an eternal glory for me that far outweighs all my problems. Let me fix my eyes on what is unseen rather than what is seen, for the seen is temporary, the unseen eternal (see 2 Corinthians 4:17-18).

Lord God, help me to not allow the worries of this life, the deceitfulness of wealth and the desires for other things come in and choke Your Word, making it unfruitful (see Mark 4:19).

Group Prayer Requests Today's Date:______________

Name	Request	Results

CLAIMING MY CALLING IN CHRIST

Week Four

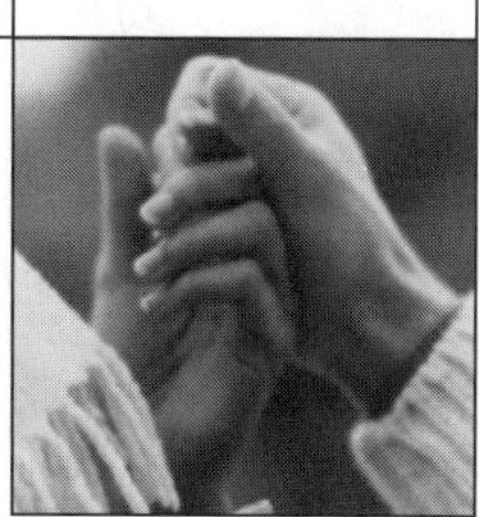

MEMORY VERSE

And over all these virtues put on love, which binds them all together in perfect unity.

Colossians 3:14

In this fourth week of the study, the time has come for you to stake your claim to your calling in Christlikeness and your claim is that God has promised to transform you into His Son's image.

This week's focus is on Christlikeness in every area of your life. The memory verse for this week emphasizes that the overarching virtue in true Christlikeness is love. Remember that memorizing God's Word will help you not only in facing temptation and handling difficult situations, but also in forming relationships and overcoming obstacles.

DAY 1: *Listening to the Shepherd's Voice*

The most difficult aspect of being Christlike may be the ability to hear Christ's voice with your heart. So many other demands often drown out the gentle voice of our loving Shepherd.

➳ What is the promise found in John 10:27-28?

eternal life, God knows us

What does it mean to hear His voice? Few believers have ever heard an audible voice like Jesus heard at His baptism, but He speaks to you in many ways. To hear His voice implies responsiveness to the Spirit's nudge in our hearts to do and be what the Spirit directs. In John 16:12-15, Jesus declares that the Holy Spirit will speak to His followers.

➳ Place a check beside the ways the Spirit has spoken to you since you became a Christian.

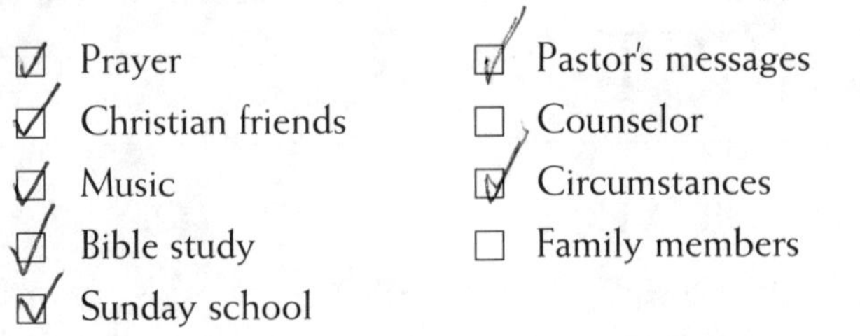

- [x] Prayer
- [x] Christian friends
- [x] Music
- [x] Bible study
- [x] Sunday school
- [x] Pastor's messages
- [ ] Counselor
- [x] Circumstances
- [ ] Family members

➳ What has been the most dramatic way the Spirit has spoken to you?

During prayer—telling me He was going to give us a baby

In John 10:11,14, Jesus stated, "I am the good shepherd."

➳ What does Jesus being your Good Shepherd mean to you?

Knows me & loves me - will take care of me.

➳ How does this fact help you listen for His guidance?

I desire His perfect will.

Knowing that Christ looks after your every need as a Good Shepherd should help you draw near to Him and allow Him to direct your life. In addition to listening for His voice, you are to claim your calling in Christ by submitting to His lordship. The spirit of joyful submission to Christ's rule must shape any activity of seeking to abound in Christ's love. In Romans 12:9, Paul insists that for those who desire to be truly Christlike, "love must be sincere" or without hypocrisy.

➳ Match the action required with the object of the action, according to Romans 12:9-11.

c	Hate	a. good.
a	Cling to	b. the Lord.
d	Honor	c. evil.
b	Serve	d. one another.

Sincere love originates in deferring to Christ's lordship and listening to His voice. This love reflects your commitment to live as Paul taught in Romans 12:9-11.

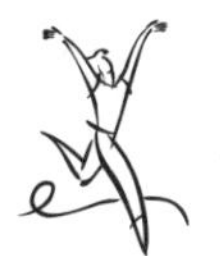

God, help me to be sincere in serving You. Help me to cling to You and to serve others.

Lord, help me to be obedient to Your voice without complaining or disputing.

DAY 2: *Receiving God's Guidance*

God knows that people, like sheep, need much direction! The Good Shepherd wants His sheep to hear His voice and follow His guidance. David observed several ways that his Shepherd King guided his life. He is also your Shepherd and will guide you in the same way.

➳ After reading Psalm 23, complete the statements below that describe ways that God guides:

- He makes me lie down in green pastures.
- He leads me beside still waters.
- He restores my soul.
- He guides me in paths of righteousness for his name's sake.
- His rod and staff comfort me.
- He prepares a table before me in the presence of my enemies.
- He ~~ant~~ anoints my head with oil.

➳ Which of the seven shepherd statements listed above means the most to you? Why?

- What does Psalm 32:8-10 promise?

  He will teach us

- How could your obedience to God be compared to a horse or a mule?

  I don't listen and obey like I should.

- What surrounds the person who trusts God?

  the Lord's love

- What does God say about His provision in Psalm 27:1-3?

  He is my stronghold

God will give you confidence and courage no matter what you are facing. Consider Psalm 37:1-7. David spelled out ways to abound in God's love.

- Mark each of the following statements either T (for true) or F (for false); then note in which verse the true ones are found:

  T Trust in the Lord and do good.
  T Commit your way to the Lord.
  F Focus your thoughts on what worldly people have.
  ? Delight yourself in God and what He gives you.
  F Set your heart on the successes of those around you.
  T Wait patiently and quietly for God to act.

Are you letting God's love abound in you as you follow the commitments you made to First Place? Are you letting God take over your fear of failure about your weight loss? Today's lesson reminds us of God's love,

His mercy and His desire to guide us in all endeavors. Call on Him today in prayer and recommit yourself to God's guidance as you keep your eye on Him.

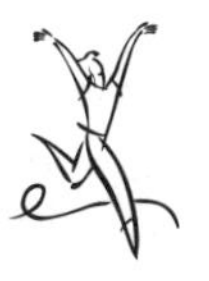

Lord, help me to acknowledge You in all areas of my life and follow Your guidance.

Oh God, I praise Your name. Be the Lord of lords and God of gods in my life.

DAY 3: *Responding to God's Discipline*

Sometimes God's guidance takes the form of discipline or correction. A Christlike life of obedience and victory requires discipline. Hebrews 12:11 promises a "harvest of righteousness" as a result of God's discipline in our lives. When you let your negative habits, such as overeating, get out of control, God will step in to correct you in a loving way that sometimes hurts.

- According to Proverbs 3:11-12, what two attitudes must be avoided when experiencing God's correction?

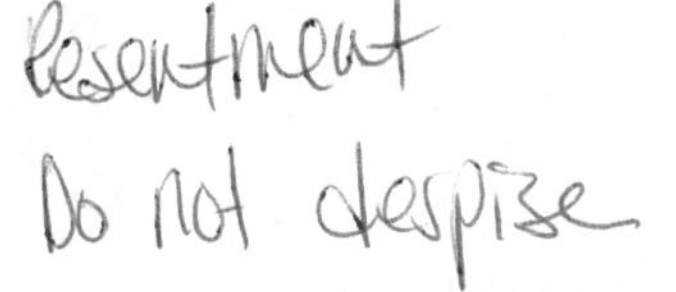

- What does God's correction prove about His regard for you?

He loves me

Just as parental discipline proves love for a child, so does God's discipline prove His love for you. You must avoid the attitude of resenting His correction or becoming weary of it. God is patient and will keep correcting you until you get it right, no matter how tired you are of hearing God's voice.

In the following four situations of persons in a First Place program, decide which ones are demonstrating a proper attitude toward discipline. Circle their names.

- Kathy is a member of a First Place group at her church. At potluck meals she always brings something with her that is within the guidelines of the Live-It plan and gladly shares with others. She is grateful for finding a way to control her eating.
- Angela is also a member of First Place and she, too, always brings First Place food with her for the potluck suppers. She constantly reminds others that she's on a diet and laments because her food isn't tasty, and she wishes she could eat like everyone else.
- Steve must eat out frequently as part of his job. He takes his Live-It plan in his billfold and carefully selects healthy items from the menu without calling attention to himself or his new eating habits. He is thankful for a plan that allows him to eat healthy even when eating out.
- Chuck also eats out frequently, but he constantly complains to his dinner companions that he's on a diet and can't eat what they do. He then makes a big show of ordering healthy foods from the menu and constantly reminds his friends that his food isn't all that tasty, but at least he's eating healthy.

Discipline in the First Place program calls for lifestyle changes. An attitude of resentment because you can't eat like everyone else will eventually affect your Bible study and prayer time. It will also cause you to find excuses not to exercise.

What does God say about discipline in Revelation 3:19?

After reading Philippians 2:1-5, correct the following statements by rewriting them:

- Focus on your own opinions and ideas.

  ____

- Seek differences with fellow believers.

  ____

- Consider ~~yourself~~ others better than ~~others~~ you.

  ____

- Insist that others do what you think is best.

  ____

- Focus on what you like because others don't know what interests them.

  ____

- Try to have the same attitude ~~that you see in others~~ as Jesus.

  ____

➳ Check the box next to any of the following actions that describe you:

- ☒ I complain to anyone who will listen.
- ☒ I accept change with gratefulness.
- ☐ I strive to keep the nine commitments that help me in being a good overseer of my body.
- ☐ I haphazardly keep the nine commitments whenever I can.

Both Psalm 37 and Philippians 2 underscore the reality that human nature does not naturally seek to abound in Christ's love. Your spirit has to be molded by His Spirit for you to overflow with His love.

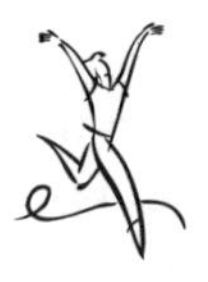

Lord, I commit myself anew today to receiving Your caring correction in all areas of my life.

Father, help me to put on love and be of one accord with You.

DAY 4: *Fulfilling God's Purpose for My Creation*

As expressed in Revelation 4:11, you were created by God and He is worthy of all the glory, honor, praise and power you can give. He created you for a purpose, for by Him all things were created.

In the following list of statements, check the box next to the one that best describes what you are doing that fulfills God's purpose for creating you:

☐ Loving Him	☐ Worshiping Him
☐ Obeying Him	☐ Sacrificing for Him
☐ Listening to Him	☐ Making changes in my life for Him

➻ What do you need to do at this point in your life to fulfill His purpose?

➻ Match the following Scripture verses with statements that express God's purpose for you:

____	Genesis 2:15	a. Live blamelessly among other people.
____	Genesis 5:24	b. Oversee what God has created.
____	Genesis 6:9	c. Become God's friend through faith.
____	Isaiah 41:8	d. Serve others for God's sake.
____	Matthew 25:40	e. Love others as you love God.
____	1 John 4:21	f. Walk continually with God.

If you are to fulfill the purpose of your creation, you must develop the characteristics of a child of God. In Ephesians 4:1-4, Paul identifies character qualities that assist the believer to achieve the goal of living "a life worthy of the calling you have received."

➻ List the five character qualities from this Scripture passage.

➻ Which of these qualities would help you to submit more completely to Christ's lordship? Explain how it would help you overcome your struggle with diet and exercise.

Today you have studied several traits and actions that can assist you in fulfilling the purpose of your creation and deferring to Christ's lordship in your life. Continue to focus on the actions of sincere love and the character qualities you want to develop, remembering to bind them all together with love.

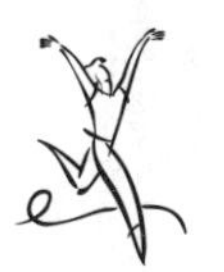

Lord, help me to develop the character traits I need to make You Lord of my life.

Father, instruct me and teach me the way I should go.

DAY 5: *Putting on Christ's Love*

Getting dressed is an important part of each day's business. More important than getting dressed physically is getting dressed spiritually by putting on Christ daily. This means to clothe yourself in the character of Christ.

What are the seven Christlike virtues listed in Colossians 3:12-13?

Look at this list of Christlike virtues and place a checkmark beside the virtues you especially need to develop in your life.

Write this week's verse from memory to show which virtue should be placed above all the rest.

Match the Scripture references with the truth each teaches about how God demonstrates His love for us.

____	Exodus 13:21	a. God loves us in spite of our sins.
____	Psalm 32:8	b. God's Spirit leads us into truth.
____	Jeremiah 31:3	c. God guides us daily.
____	Hosea 3:1	d. God treats us with loving kindness.
____	John 16:13	e. God teaches us how to live.
____	Romans 8:39	f. God's love overcomes all circumstances.

Being a Christian is more than your personal love relationship with Jesus. God wants you to put on His love each day by loving others sacrificially, just as Jesus lay down His life for you. Claiming your calling in Christ requires you to love God supremely and to love others as you love yourself.

Have you remembered to call or write group members this week to encourage them? Have you demonstrated God's love in your everyday life? Accept the challenge and show God's love to others through your own actions.

Lord, pour Your Holy Spirit into me and make me a vessel worthy of the prize You have set for me.

Lord, help me to put on Your love each day and clothe myself with Christlike virtues.

DAY 6: *Reflections*

During this week's study you have learned more about the characteristics unique to Christ. You have been challenged to develop the discipline of abounding love. If you find loving and accepting others difficult, that may be a stronghold keeping you from your full blessing in Jesus. Being unable to forgive someone else for a hurt done to you also can become a stronghold and keep you from success in reaching your goals.

Memorizing the memory verse as well as other verses of Scripture will help you in praying for a specific area of your life. God gives you a divine weapon to fight the hurt and sense of failure you may experience in trying to live your life as He would have you live.

The Scripture Memory Music CDs are an excellent resource to help you memorize. Writing down the memory verse in your prayer journal or on your Commitment Record will help you familiarize yourself with the words. Repeat them several times in a row until you can say the words easily.

As you pray today, use the following Scriptures as examples. Memorize the verses; then take advantage of them when you pray for guidance in loving others.

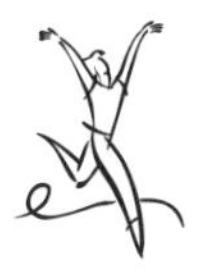

Dear Lord, help me to love not with just words or my tongue but with my actions and in truth because You have loved me (see 1 John 3:18).

Lord, help me to love others; for love comes from You; and everyone that loves is born of You and knows You. Help me to always remember that You are love (see 1 John 4:7-8).

Heavenly Father, let my love be sincere. Let me hate what is evil and cling only to what is good. Let me be kindly towards others with brotherly love; honoring others before myself (see Romans 12:9-10).

DAY 7: *Reflections*

This week's study has focused on your calling in Christ. God created you for a purpose. He has given you an overflowing attitude of kindness in your everyday life. He has shown His love for you through His death on the Cross. As you listen to your Shepherd's voice, let Him guide you to fulfilling His purpose in you. Respond to His discipline in a positive way that will lead you to accepting His lordship in your life.

If you attempt to follow through with your nine commitments to First Place without God's help, you will find failure comes quickly. Using Scriptures relevant to your situation, you will find God's help easily accessible as you pray for Him to help you. Keeping the commitments is in direct relationship to a spirit of joyful submission to God's rule in your life.

In review of what was said last week: Memorizing Scripture will help you handle difficult situations, overcome temptation and give you guidance. Praying through Scripture—personalizing the verse by putting your name in key places and translating it into your own language will help you gain ownership over the verse.

Each week's study includes verses you can use as you learn to pray through the Scriptures. Once you become accustomed to this method of praying, find verses of your own and use them in your prayers.

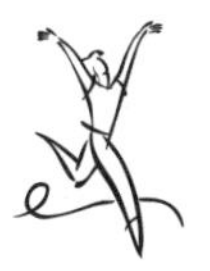

O Lord, I know that all things work together for good because I love You and am called to Your purpose (see Romans 8:28).

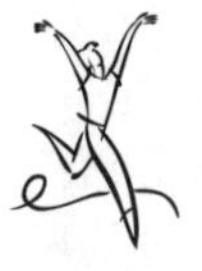

Lord, I know I have been justified through faith and I can have peace with You through my Lord Jesus Christ through whom I have access by faith to Your grace (see Romans 5:1-2).

Heavenly Father, over all the virtues I have through You, let me put on love which binds us all together in perfect unity (see Colossians 3:14).

Group Prayer Requests Today's Date:______________

Name	Request	Results

RUNNING FOR THE PRIZE

Week Five

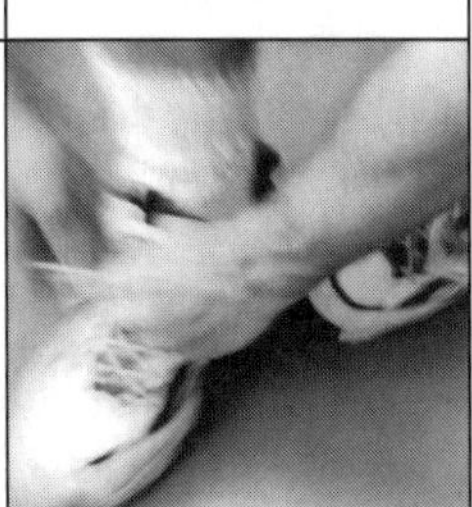

MEMORY VERSE

But you, man of God, flee from all of this,
and pursue righteousness, godliness, faith,
love, endurance and gentleness.
1 Timothy 6:11

You are now at the halfway point in this session. We pray you are still pressing on toward your goal to win the prize for which God has called you heavenward in Christ Jesus (see Philippians 3:14). In 1 Corinthians 9:24, Paul states, "Run in such a way as to get the prize." This means that you must do those things in First Place which will help you reach your goal. When you keep the nine commitments, you are doing your best to obtain the prize.

This week's memory verse describes the prize before us. Paul was warning Timothy to flee materialism and pursue character traits leading to intimate fellowship with God, like a runner seeking a prize. Last week's lesson about being Christlike can be applied as you press on to intimate fellowship with Him.

DAY 1: *The Motivation for the Race*

After many years of relentless and faithful pursuit of the prize, Paul challenged Timothy (in 1 Timothy 6:11) to be in hot pursuit of the character qualities that enhance intimate fellowship with God. He went on (in verse 12) to encourage him to "fight the good fight of the faith."

Paul coached Timothy on having a winning attitude. Winning a championship is a very important achievement for any athletic team. Some observers believe that what sets a championship team apart is their eagerness to win rather than their fear of failure. The world needs the witness of Christians who reflect the eagerness and confidence of sports champions.

Such enthusiasm causes others to want to run with you. Being faithful in that witness is an important part of the race for the prize.

Just as motivation is important for the athlete, it is important for you in First Place.

- Which of the following motivations inspire you to victories in your Christian life? Rank them according to their importance in your experience with 1 being the most important and 6 being the least.

____	Thankfulness	____	Forgiveness
____	Prayer	____	Worship
____	Victories	____	Service

- Record an experience in which God used one of these motivations to accomplish a significant victory over a menacing spiritual foe.

In 1 John 2:15-17, John warned his readers to flee worldly lures and focus on eternal values.

- What should be our motivation in spiritual pursuits?

- Fill in the missing words from 1 John 2:17.

The ____________________ and its __________________ pass ____________________, but the man who __________ the will of __________________ lives __________________.

Romans 5:3-4 demonstrates how perseverance takes the believer from suffering to hope.

- Number the following words in the order Paul lists them in these verses:

____	Character	____	Perseverance
____	Suffering	____	Hope

- How have you seen the process of moving from suffering to perseverance to character to hope occur in your own life?

- Write a sentence thanking God for the determination of endurance He is accomplishing in you in one of the following areas:

Marriage	Spiritual growth	Financial security
Health needs	Emotional stability	Personal well-being
Healthy eating	Exercise	Weight loss

Eagerness and determination go together. The overall goal of First Place is to put God first in our lives. Our eagerness to do God's will for our lives will motivate us to keep our commitments and press on to our goals. A love relationship with God should give us an eagerness for Christian living. Ask God for a zest for the task and an eagerness for running in a way that will help you obtain your prize. As others sense your spirit of eagerness, they, too, will be encouraged to run life's race for Christ.

Becoming Christlike is a long-term process, and no believer experiences only victories in the Christian life.

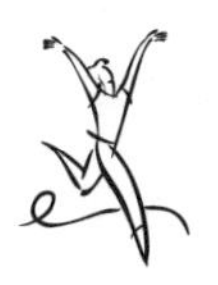

Lord, give me the patience I need to endure setbacks and help me set my eyes on the prize You have set before me.

DAY 2: *The Rigors of Righteousness*

With the same intensity as an Olympic hopeful training for a medal, God's children must pursue righteousness.

- According to Mark 12:30-31, how are we to love God? How are we to love our neighbors?

- What does 1 John 4:10-12 tell us about loving God and our neighbors?

The whole law of God is based on love. Righteousness involves living in balance by relating properly to God and others. Righteousness demonstrates itself through distinctive behavior.

- What specific actions could you take to obey God's command?

The Scriptures tell us to "be still, and know that I am God" (Psalm 46:10). Step out of your comfort zone. Follow Jesus' example for a balanced life. When running for the prize of fellowship with God, we must run full throttle with exuberance and excellence. The determination to endure insures that we will reach the prize—intimate fellowship with God. If you love God above all else, you will have an intimate relationship with Him, and you will love others as God loves you.

- Hebrews 12:1-2 tells us how we must run the race that God has set before us. In your own words, describe how we must run our race.

➳ At what points in Jesus' life could He have given up?

➳ Why didn't He give up?

Since your faith begins and ends in Jesus, and you are surrounded by so many witnesses, you must do everything you can to run with endurance the race set before you.

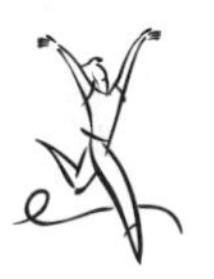

Lord, give me the strength I need each day to run the race and persevere to the end.

Father God, thank You for loving me and enduring the pain of the Cross.

DAY 3: *The Goodness of Godliness*

Godliness is godlikeness; Paul emphasized godliness in his first letter to Timothy. He associates godliness with several important qualities or characteristics.

➳ Read the following verses in 1 Timothy; then match each one with the quality or action described by it:

____	2:1-2	a. The goodness of creation
____	4:4	b. Contentment
____	4:7	c. Godly training
____	6:3	d. Pray for leaders
____	6:6	e. Sound instruction and godly teaching

- Which of these godly characteristics seems to be most present in your life?

- How do you cultivate this quality?

- Read 2 Peter 1:3-7. Between which two qualities does the word "godliness" appear in verses 6 and 7?

- What are some examples of these two characteristics in your relationships with others?

- How have these two qualities helped you grow in godliness?

Gentleness is another quality that the believer pursues in his or her quest for the prize of intimate fellowship with God.

- Describe how the gentleness of Jesus is illustrated in the following two passages:

  - Matthew 11:28-30

  - Mark 10:14-16

Jesus models gentleness of spirit for all of His followers. We are to daily reflect Christ's gentleness and humility.

➳ How does Matthew 21:5 illustrate humility?

Godliness nourishes the soul. Those born again in Christ must not forfeit anything that is necessary to live a life of godliness in Him. In spite of all the worldliness about us, we must press on for the prize by developing the attributes of godliness.

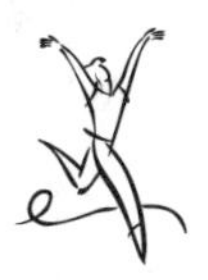

Dear Lord, give me a gentle, loving spirit as I follow the path that will lead me to the prize of godliness.

Father, help me to cultivate the characteristics I need to be a godly witness for You.

DAY 4: *The Victory of Faith*

The victory of faith results in the blessings of regular fellowship with God. The New Testament gives many examples of faith's victory. This victory comes from trusting God instead of caving in to circumstances. What could be more encouraging than reviewing the victory of faith?

➳ Match the following passages with Paul's teaching:

____	2 Corinthians 5:7	a. We are justified by faith.
____	Galatians 3:24	b. We are shielded by faith.
____	Ephesians 6:16	c. We must walk by faith.

We must demonstrate our faith by the way we live it out.

➳ What does Ephesians 2:8 mean to you?

Grace through faith supplies the gift of salvation. Other New Testament writers also praised faith's victory.

➳ Match verses with the correct phrases about faith.

____	Matthew 17:20	a. Faith overcomes the world.
____	Hebrews 11:1	b. Faith pleases God.
____	Hebrews 11:6	c. With faith nothing is impossible.
____	1 John 5:4	d. Faith means being sure of what we hope for.

What testimonies these writers have given to the power of faith. If you press on in faith instead of fear, you can face the issues and concerns that come into your life. Spend time every day with God. Read His Word and talk to Him who gives you life.

➳ The following Scripture passages provide a picture of the role faith played in the lives of several people who encountered Jesus. Read the Scripture; then explain how each person exhibited faith.

- Jairus (Mark 5:22-24,35-43)

- The woman with an issue of blood (Mark 5:25-34)

- The blind man (Mark 10:46-52)

- The sinful woman (Luke 7:36-38,44-50)

These are but four examples from a multitude of followers of Jesus who demonstrated their faith and were healed.

➳ What are ways you have exhibited faith in God?

Exercise your faith this week as you rely on God to help you press on to your goal and reach the prize.

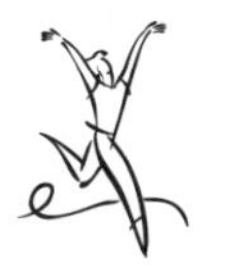

Lord, help me to demonstrate my faith in You because I know faith in You is the evidence of things not seen.

Father, thank You for Your gift of grace through Jesus because I live by faith in the Son of God.

DAY 5: *The Face of Love*

As we pursue intimate fellowship with God, we must continually remind ourselves that He looks on us through eyes of love. Many believers see God more with the face of a demanding taskmaster than with the face of a loving father. To them, God looks like a divine accountant regularly sending another statement to remind us that we still owe Him.

- After reading Luke 22:59-62, check the following statement that most accurately reflects what you think Jesus felt when He looked at Peter's face after Peter denied Him:

  - ☐ Revulsion because Peter behaved so cowardly.
  - ☐ Pity that Peter would miss such a witnessing opportunity.
  - ☐ Compassion toward Peter in spite of his denial.
  - ☐ Satisfaction because His prophecy about Peter was correct.

- How does Jesus' treatment of Peter in John 21:15-19 encourage you when you feel you have failed Him?

In last week's study we learned that God wants us to demonstrate His love each day by loving others. First Corinthians 13—the love chapter—paints the best portrait of the face of love in the Bible.

- Match the positive characteristics of love listed with the actions that illustrate each quality.

____ Patient	1. Looking out for the safety of children
____ Kind	2. Following God despite setbacks
____ Rejoices	3. Visiting a friend in the hospital
____ Protects	4. Accepting another's decision on a problem
____ Trusts	5. Waiting on God to open up a way
____ Hopes	6. Daring to believe in the face of obstacles
____ Perseveres	7. Celebrating a friend's promotion

- Which of the seven actions sounds most like you?

- Which of the actions are easiest for you?

- Which may be a problem for you? Why?

- What does Solomon have to say about gentleness in Proverbs 15:1?

- What truth about gentleness is revealed in 1 Peter 3:3-4?

Soft answers to another's anger and a gentle witness enable Christians to have maximum impact on those with whom they come into contact. As you experience more of His love toward you, you can regularly show His love to others. His love will flow through you in such a way that you become a testimony of God's love and you will be identified as His child.

Are you demonstrating God's love in your everyday life? Make a phone call to a member or your leader, share the memory verse with a friend or send a note of encouragement to someone who needs a lift or a kind word from a Christian friend.

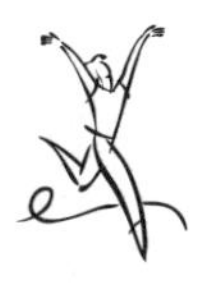

Lord, let Your love shine through me so that others may see You in me.

Heavenly Father, give me the strength to turn away anger with a soft answer.

DAY 6: *Reflections*

During this week's study you have learned more about God's love and gentleness. The memory verse for this week reminds us of the traits we are to develop in our race for the prize. Being like Christ means to endure the rigors of righteousness, experience the goodness of godliness, love, be gentle and have faith as we press on toward our goal.

The power of prayer gives us the strength to endure the race as we openly seek God's will and purpose in our lives. Prayer will give us determination and the support we need to fight the strongholds that come in and cause us to stumble. Whether your stronghold is unhealthy eating, a schedule too busy for Bible study or exercise, a lack of faith in God to do what He promised or an unforgiving spirit, prayer using Scripture can knock down the walls and set you free to reach your goals.

As you pray today, use the following Scriptures as examples. Memorize the verses; then use them when you pray for endurance to finish the race.

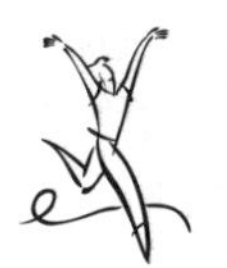

Lord, You have forgiven me for so much. Make it evident in the way I love You and love others (see Luke 7:47).

Heavenly Father, I have heard the world say that I should love my neighbor and hate my enemy, but You tell me to love my enemies and pray for those who persecute me, that I might be a child of You, my Father in heaven. Help me to love like You (see Matthew 5:43-44).

Lord God, I know You are my sun and shield, and I pray for Your grace and glory to be evident in my life, for I know You do not withhold any good thing from me when I walk blamelessly (see Psalm 84:11).

DAY 7: *Reflections*

This week's study has focused on the pursuit of those traits that will help us reach the goal we have set for ourselves. Our prize is intimate relationship with God.

Sometimes things of the world come in and try to steer us off course. This is when we need the Scriptures we have memorized to keep us on the right track. Remember the Scripture from week three that warns about those things that come into your life and choke out the Word? When a desire for wealth and other things choke out the Word, your life becomes unfruitful. Remember how Jesus used Scripture to fight Satan during His days in the wilderness (see Matthew 4:1-11)? When your own wilderness comes, you will have the verses you need to bring you out of temptation and trouble.

If you are still having a problem memorizing verses, try breaking them down into two or three words at a time, thinking about their meaning then adding phrase by phrase. Repetition is the easiest way to memorize. Say the verse over and over to yourself during the day using the Scripture memory book.

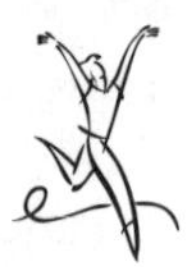

Father God, if I love those who love me, what reward will I get? Are not even the godless doing that? And if I greet only those whom I like, what am I doing more than others? Even pagans do that. You have called me to be different, Lord! You have called me to go far beyond the actions of even the noblest pagan (see Matthew 5:46-47).

Heavenly Father, help me to bear much fruit so as to be a disciple who will glorify You through my faith (see John 15:8).

Lord, You have told me that I am to present my body as a living sacrifice, holy, acceptable to You. I am not to be conformed to this world, but transformed by the renewing of my mind that I may prove what is that good and acceptable and perfect will of God. I offer up my body as a living sacrifice, a testament of Your mercy (see Romans 12:1-2).

Heavenly Father, help me to flee from all sin and pursue righteousness, godliness, faith, love, endurance and gentleness (see 1 Timothy 6:11).

Group Prayer Requests Today's Date:________________

Name	Request	Results

TRAINING FOR THE RACE

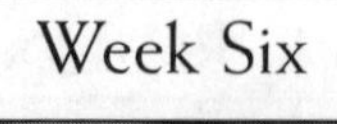

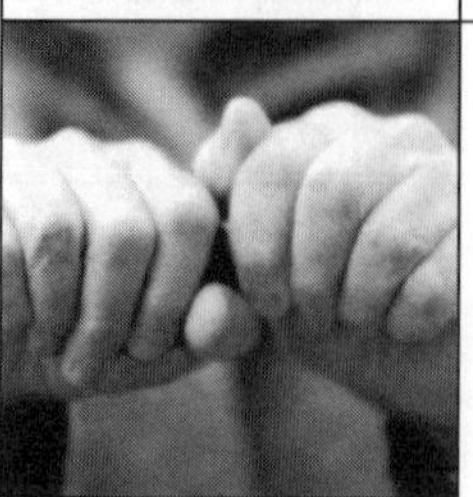

MEMORY VERSE

Do you not know that in a race
all the runners run, but only one gets the prize?
Run in such a way as to get the prize.
1 Corinthians 9:24

Games create a certain mania wherever and whenever they are played. The Olympic Games, begun in 776 B.C., dominated the Greek culture and provided the background for much of Paul's teaching about the importance of training for daily Christian living.

This week's study encourages devotion to winning the full prize God desires for us—intimate fellowship with Him. For God's glory, with full dedication to training for the race, we press on!

DAY 1: *Train to Win*

Just as Olympic athletes train for years to earn their place on the Olympic team, Christians train to reach an intimate relationship with God. Many times they overlook the importance of training and the fact that not everyone wins. Only those who persevere and endure the rigors gain the prize. The wonderful part of being a Christian is that more than one *will* obtain the prize. Any Christian who persistently studies Scripture, prays and seeks the fellowship of Christ will gain the reward of intimate fellowship.

- Paraphrase the question posed by Paul in this week's memory verse, 1 Corinthians 9:24.

Many believers feel they are simply called to endure this life since Christ won their salvation on the cross. Salvation is the starting point, but there is much more to be won. Winning that prize requires a disciplined life.

Our focus should be doing our best, and when we see the face of Jesus at the finish line, we want to see His look of approval.

- What is the reason Paul gave for running the race?

In 1 Corinthians 9:25, it says that competitors need strict training to win the prize. The difference between you and the runner in an Olympic race is that your prize is imperishable, but the Olympic runner's prize is perishable and fades away.

- How does participation in the First Place program relate to strict training?

Losing weight is not the only goal of First Place. Study the nine commitments and you find that the mental, emotional and spiritual as well as physical needs are met. The Bible study, Scripture memory, exercise, encouragement of others and sensible eating all work together to give you success. Because you are not perfect, you will find times that you stumble and fall, but let God pick you up and set you on the right course. Don't give up because you can't follow all the commitments right away.

If ice-skater Tara Lipinski, gymnast Mary Lou Retton or speed-skater Eric Heiden had quit when they fell or didn't win a particular event, the world may never have witnessed the triumphant moment when each of them in turn stood on the Olympic Games winner's platform and had the honor of wearing the gold medal. In the words of Winston Churchill, "Never give in, never give in, never, never, never, never—in nothing, great or small, large or petty—never give in except to convictions of honour and good sense."[1]

- After reading 2 Timothy 2:3-7, number the following statements in the order Paul wrote them to Timothy:

____ Endure hardship like a good soldier.
____ Wait patiently like a good farmer.
____ Follow the rules like a good athlete.

Leave nothing undone that could contribute to victory and do away with anything that could lead to defeat. Let Proverbs 3:6 be your guide as you train: "In all your ways acknowledge him, and he will make your paths straight."

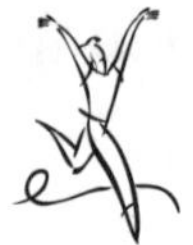

You, Lord, have declared that You know the plans You have for me. Your plans are to prosper me and not to harm me, plans to give me hope and a future. Because of all You've done for me through Your Son, Jesus, when I call upon You and come and pray to You, You will listen. I will seek You and find You when I seek You with all my heart. You have declared, "I will be found by you." You will bring me back from captivity (see Jeremiah 29:11-14).[2]

DAY 2: *Run to Win*

On the cross Christ won your salvation. His victory over sin—your salvation—is not the prize you are running for because only Christ could win that for you. Your salvation is assured; you can't earn it. However, there is a prize you can win with His help—the prize of intimate fellowship with God. Winning this prize requires strict training. Many will run the race, but not all will gain the prize of intimate fellowship. In order to win the prize, believers must not lose their focus or quit the course.

- What things can cause you to lose focus—to take your eyes off the prize?

- How can you make sure you keep your focus?

- According to Hebrews 12:1-2, what should you be fixing your eyes on?

- What are the areas in which you are seeking to follow Jesus' model for pleasing God?

- In your own words tell how Galatians 6:9-10 encourages you.

- List some specific ways in which you could serve other believers.

Winning the prize of intimate fellowship with God must be the single-minded focus of every believer. With eternal salvation secure in Christ, believers have the opportunity to live with full-throttled devotion to God.

In your efforts to keep the commitment of encouraging others, consider Ephesians 4:29. Let words that encourage, build up and edify proceed from your mouth. Just as an athlete responds to the encouragement from fans, a friend in First Place will appreciate words of encouragement from you.

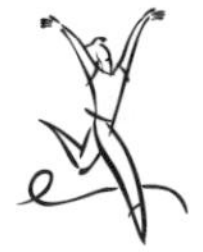

Lord, let all bitterness, anger, clamor and evil speaking be put away so that my words encourage and lift up others. Let me forgive others even as You have forgiven me.

Father God, help me to walk in Your Spirit and not be tempted by lusts of the flesh which will take me off course as I run the race.

DAY 3: *Train to Win*

Winning races requires strenuous training. As you participate in First Place, you may learn that diligent exercise allows you to lose weight and build stamina to do your daily activities. Both these benefits require that you exercise on a regular basis. Training includes stretching, toning and practice. Many exercise terms may also apply to the spiritual life.

➳ Match the following exercise terms with the correct descriptions:

____ Stretching	a. Strength built up over time
____ Toning	b. Continual regular repetition
____ Endurance	c. Extension beyond usual limitations
____ Practice	d. Small slow-paced movements

➳ From Galatians 5:22-23, list the fruit of the Spirit.

➳ How will you use spiritual stretching, toning, endurance and practice this week to develop one expression of the fruit of the Spirit?

Believers sometimes neglect spiritual training just as athletes might with physical training. For believers, the key to winning is repenting of spiritual lapses and returning to spiritual training.

➳ In Psalm 51:10-12, what did David request from God in order to be renewed in His service?

David knew the key to winning spiritually would be for God to grant the requests of his heart. Winning requires strict training. Just as your physical body needs exercise, your spirit needs spiritual exercise as you pursue the prize of intimate fellowship with God. David recognized this and asked for a return of his spiritual joy.

- According to 1 Corinthians 9:27, what was Paul's greatest fear in running the race?

Paul didn't fear losing his salvation, but he did fear disqualification from winning the prize of intimate fellowship with God. He knew that temptation could test him sorely and could cause him to get off course. No runner wants to think about being disqualified after months, or even years, of training. The prize before you outshines any temptations around us, so press on.

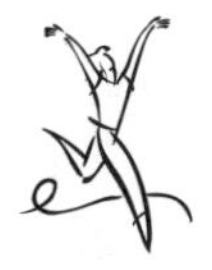

Father God, forgive me for giving in to temptations that could deter me from my set course.

Heavenly Father, I ask for the Holy Spirit to bring every condition and desire of my body into complete submission to Christ.

DAY 4: *Aim for the Goal*

An athlete's training for the race includes mental as well as physical conditioning. If he or she loses mental focus while running, all of his or her physical training will have been in vain. Perhaps Paul observed this connection among athletes of his own day.

- According to 1 Corinthians 9:24-26, what two purposes did Paul keep in mind as he ran?

➳ In Hebrews 12:2, what was the example set by Jesus?

➳ What should be the Christian's ultimate goal?

With his purposes clearly in mind, Paul could count on the provision Jesus had made for him and all of His followers by sending the Holy Spirit.

➳ What does John 16:13-15 mean to you as you run the race and seek the prize?

Jesus had complete confidence in the Holy Spirit to guide believers when they need greater understanding.

➳ Consider Galatians 5:19-23—what area of control over your body and your desires is the most difficult for you?

➳ How have you experienced God giving you a victory over the flesh by developing the fruit of the Spirit in you?

Only the Holy Spirit can bring every condition and desire of the body into complete submission to Christ.

➳ Match the following Scriptures with the truth they teach about the ministry of the Holy Spirit:

____ John 14:17	a. He tells you spiritual truths.
____ John 14:26	b. He gives directions for specific acts.
____ John 16:18	c. He lives with you and in you.
____ Acts 8:29	d. He convicts you of guilt.
____ 1 Corinthians 2:13	e. He reminds you of what Jesus said.

These actions of the Holy Spirit guide you, so you can run your race with confidence. You can boldly aim for the goal, equipped with all the spiritual resources you need to win.

Heading in the right direction is as important as running well if you want to win. A good athlete recovered a big fumble in the 1929 Rose Bowl football game, but Roy Riegels became famous not because he recovered the fumble and ran it all the way to the two-yard line. He is remembered because he made a long run to the wrong goal! It could happen to any one of us unless the Holy Spirit guides and helps us to keep our eyes on the right goal.

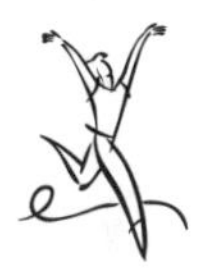

Lord, let me reap the fruit of the Spirit by helping me to love, to have joy and peace, to be patient, kind, good, faithful, gentle and self-controlled because by living in the Spirit, I will walk with the Spirit.

Father, thank You for sending the Holy Spirit to bring the desires of my body into complete submission to You.

DAY 5: *Watch Out for Wasted Effort*

Sometimes those who suit up only warm up. They practice, but they never play in the game. First Place members who come to the first few meetings and then drop out because they see no progress, cheat themselves of the fellowship with others, fellowship with God through Bible study and the prayers and encouragement of others. Stay in the game, play to the end; and the final score may be better than you think.

Paul did not run aimlessly, nor did he waste efforts by just beating the air. Paul draws illustrations from the sport of boxing. He must have observed several muscular athletes who looked like world champions warming up, but when it came to boxing toe-to-toe with a fierce opponent, they seldom landed a winning blow. How can you be sure you are not merely beating the air in your daily living? The Holy Spirit comes to our rescue by giving eternal impact to our efforts.

➳ After reading Ephesians 5:15-20, complete each of the following sentences with its correct phrase:

____ Be very careful	a. with the Holy Spirit.
____ Make the most	b. how you live.
____ Do not get drunk	c. with spiritual songs.
____ Be filled	d. on wine.
____ Speak to one another	e. to God for everything.
____ Always give thanks	f. of every opportunity.

Of all these actions, the command to be filled with the Spirit deserves priority.

➳ The following are some of the evidences of a Spirit-filled life. Put a check by those you feel you are achieving now. Put a star by those in which you may need more growth.

- ☐ Desire for spiritual growth
- ☐ Feel convicted of sin
- ☐ Enjoy fellowship with God
- ☐ Look for ways to serve God
- ☐ Seek to please God
- ☐ Love other Christians as brothers

➳ What is lacking for you to be completely filled? Check all that apply.

- ☐ I don't like to change.
- ☐ I'm doing okay as I am.
- ☐ It requires too much discipline.
- ☐ I get sidetracked by other demands.
- ☐ Other ________________________________

In Galatians 5:13-18, Paul expressed a concern that the Galatians use their freedom in Christ to serve others in love, rather than as a license for allowing the desires of the flesh to rule.

➳ In verses 16-18 Paul spells out four conditions that produce four results. Match the condition on the left with the result on the right.

____	Live by the Spirit.	a. You do not do what you want.
____	If led by the Spirit.	b. You are not under law.
____	They are in conflict.	c. The Spirit opposes sin nature.
____	Sin nature opposes the Spirit.	d. Don't gratify the sinful nature.

When you live your life without depending completely on the Holy Spirit, you waste effort and beat the air. Fight to win. Put on the armor and face the enemy. The Holy Spirit knows the will of God completely and will keep you from merely beating the air.

Father God, help me to follow the Spirit fully as I seek to press on toward the prize.

Lord, give me the strength I need to run the race and be in complete submission to You.

Day 6: *Reflections*

Paul delivers a very strong statement about the toughest area to conquer when training one's own body. The body itself needs continual discipline if you are to win a spiritual prize. Scripture memory and prayer are the most powerful tools you have to fight the strongholds in life that attempt to defeat your efforts.

Sometimes past failures and bad experiences come to mind and make you feel like you should be disqualified from the prize of intimate fellowship with God. God can help you claim His forgiveness and cleansing. His Word contains many teachings on forgiveness. Allowing any stronghold from the past or present to come in and choke out the Word of God will cause you pain.

As you use the Scripture Memory Music CD and *Walking in the Word* book to learn the memory verses, think of how you can use the Scripture as a prayer.

Pray today using the following Scriptures as examples. Memorize the verses then take advantage of them when you pray for the endurance to finish the race.

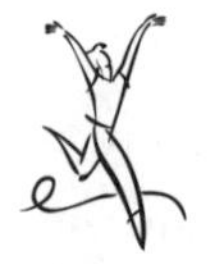

Lord, help me to be more like You. You are forgiving and good, O Lord, abounding in love to all who call to You (see Psalm 86:5).

Father, You made me; You will sustain me and You will rescue me. You are God, and there is no other; You are God, and there is none like You (see Isaiah 46:4,9).

Father God, give me a humble spirit and forbid me from boasting except in the cross of my Lord Jesus Christ, by whom the world has been crucified to me and I to the world (see Galatians 6:14).

DAY 7: *Reflections*

This week's study focused on running the race in such a way as to win the prize of intimacy with Jesus. Review this week's memory verse—1 Corinthians 9:24. Paul commands that we run to get the prize. He closed chapter 9 by underscoring his concern for running for the prize in such a way as to avoid being disqualified.

Memorizing and using Scriptures will help you in running the race successfully. With God's Word as your guide, you will not face disqualification. Scripture memory helps to discipline your mind just as you run and discipline your body. Claim the promises of God and renew your commitment to run for the prize. The prize of intimate fellowship with God is more valuable than any treasure that man could conceive. It is yours if you desire it, but you must discipline your mind and body in such a way as to win.

When temptations come, no matter what their form, memorized Scripture helps you face and overcome them because God's Word gives you the power needed to win.

Lord God, help me to not be overcome by evil, but to overcome evil with good (see Romans 12:21).

Blessed am I because my transgressions are forgiven. Blessed am I because my sins are covered. May my deep gratitude be evident in the way I relate to others, O Lord (see Psalm 32:1).

Heavenly Father, You are my light and salvation, and I have nothing to fear. Though the enemy may encamp about me, my heart shall not fear. Give me the courage to fight my strongholds unafraid so that I may dwell in house of the Lord all of my days (see Psalm 27:1,3-4).

Lord, I know all the runners run in a race and only one gets the prize. Help me to run in such a way that I will win the prize (see 1 Corinthians 9:24).

Notes

1. Winston Churchill, in a speech at Harrow School, October 29, 1941.
2. Beth Moore, *Praying God's Word* (Nashville, TN: Broadman and Holman, 2000), p. 124.

Group Prayer Requests Today's Date:______________

Name	Request	Results

RECEIVING AN EVERLASTING CROWN

Week Seven

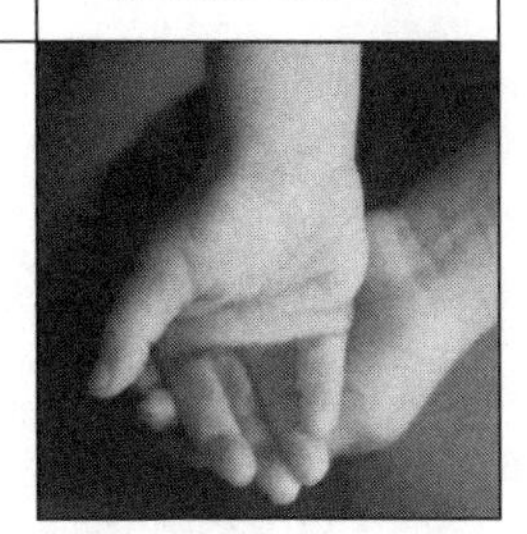

MEMORY VERSE

And when the Chief Shepherd appears,
you will receive the crown of glory
that will never fade away.
1 Peter 5:4

In the Olympic Games, three victors stand on the podium and receive their medals from a member of the awards committee. The crowds cheer, the flags rise to the top and a band plays the national anthem. Spectators see the smiles and tears of joy on the faces of champions who stand tall because they have given their best. This is repeated over and over again for each athletic competition.

Imagine a similar scene in heaven as believers kneel before the King. They receive the crown of glory from God Himself because they have kept the faith, endured the race, walked with the Lord and achieved intimate fellowship with Him. Heavenly music rings out and angels sing the glory and honor of God. Those who have gone before rejoice at the new crowns being given. In the worldly competition only one can receive the prize, but in the heavenly race all who achieve the goal will win the prize of intimate fellowship with God and will wear that crown of life! Wow! Does that give you goose bumps?

This week's study focuses on the challenge to win the prize, which is sometimes called the crown of life. The memory verse reminds us to live our lives ever mindful of an everlasting prize—the crown of glory. Run to win so that for all eternity you can claim the prize of intimate fellowship with God.

DAY 1: *Two Different Crowns*

In 1 Corinthians 9:24 Paul insisted, "Run in such a way as to get the prize." In the first part of verse 25, Paul encouraged strict training. He concluded with an observation about athletes.

➳ Why does an athlete run in a race?

➳ Why do Christians run the race?

David and his son Absalom also wore crowns. David wore his crown legitimately, but Absalom wore his illegitimately.

➳ After reading 1 Samuel 16:1-13, consider verse 7. What was God's command to Samuel as he looked at Jesse's sons?

➳ What does this mean to you as you follow your commitments to First Place?

Outward appearances fade in importance when God looks on the heart. He requires a pure heart focused on Him. Samuel was uncertain, but he followed God's direction and anointed David. David never forgot that God chose him and gave him the crown that he wore as king. David was a man after God's own heart (see 1 Samuel 13:14; Acts 13:22).

Consider 2 Samuel 15:6-12 and how different Absalom's rise to become king was.

➳ Mark the following responses T (for true) or F (for false):

____ Absalom publicly announced his plans to be the king.
____ Absalom used trumpets to proclaim the beginning of his rule.
____ Absalom let his closest friends know about his plans.
____ Absalom recruited his father's advisor to help him.

____ Absalom's conspiracy grew stronger the longer it went.

____ Absalom gained his father's blessing to become king.

God gave David his crown. Absalom took his crown by popularity and force. David's crown represents an everlasting crown that only God can give. Absalom's crown represents a temporary crown that people will give and take as they please.

- According to 2 Samuel 18:6-15, Absalom used secrecy and underhandedness to take away his father's crown. What happened to Absalom?

- What are the consequences when someone wins a prize for the wrong reasons or with the wrong motives?

David and Absalom represent two very different types of crowns. Each crown stands for the different goal that people strive for in life. Eternity will reveal to all which crown has greater value.

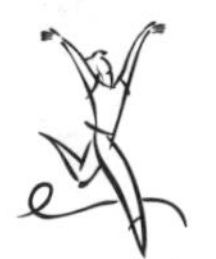

God, give me the desire and endurance to pursue the prize of the everlasting crown.

DAY 2: *The Crown of Life and Rejoicing*

The purpose for living is to win the prize God has for us—intimate fellowship with Him. In 1 Corinthians 9:25, Paul referred to this prize as the everlasting crown.

In James 1:3-12, James stated that the one who endures the test will receive the crown of life that God has promised. Paul's everlasting crown and James's crown of life are the same. The believer running for the prize receives this crown from God. James instructed the believers in advance to expect to face many kinds of tests.

- What is the blessing in verse 12 and who is to receive the crown?

- Describe a test or temptation you feel you have endured. What was the result?

- Write a prayer to God expressing a need you currently have. Use a Scripture passage that has special meaning to you for this need.

In Revelation, John recorded Christ's triumphant words to believers to hang on through trials to receive the crown of life. Read Revelation 2:8-10, where Christ challenged the believers in Smyrna to remain faithful, promising He would reward them.

- Place a check mark next to any of the following words that identify some of the conditions believers would have to endure:

☐ Afflictions	☐ Immorality
☐ Prison	☐ Poverty
☐ Earthquakes	☐ Slander

- What was their reward?

- What has helped you get through your trials and hardships?

Jesus, James and Paul all taught about the wonderful gift of the crown of life. Focusing on the crown must sustain us when the trials of life bring us down.

- Considering 1 Thessalonians 2:19-20, what is your hope, joy or crown?

Paul may be referring to both evangelism and Christian brotherhood as parts of the everlasting crown that we receive from God. Pursuing the prize of intimate fellowship with God produces results in other areas of our lives. We will be winning people to Christ and cultivating meaningful relationships with them in God's family.

- After reading John 15:1-8, list two reasons Jesus says we are to bear much fruit.

Bearing much fruit brings glory to the heavenly Father and shows that we are Christ's disciples. Consider Isaiah 35:10; although the promise will be consummated in heaven, it still applies to believers on Earth.

- When was the last time you felt overtaken by the joy of God?

Many choirs and churches sing the anthem, "Crown Him with many crowns, the Lamb upon the throne." What a glorious day that will be when each believer is crowned with a crown of life by the One who sits upon the throne of heaven. Then all your hard work, endurance, patience, love and faithfulness will be worth every effort you put forth to achieve the prize, and you will reign with Him throughout eternity.

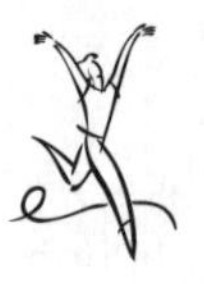

Father God, help me to be faithful through good times and the hard times so that I may receive the crown of life.

Lord, restore to me the joy of my salvation and let me rejoice and praise Your name.

DAY 3: *The Crown of Righteousness and Worship*

The eternal crown from God includes the crown of righteousness and the crown of worship. The crown of righteousness emphasizes our relationship to God. God bestows it on those who give priority to intimately relating to Him. The crown of worship is all the crowns combined in the everlasting crown.

- After reading 2 Timothy 4:6-8, draw a line to complete the sentences with the correct phrases.

I have fought	the race.
I have finished	the faith.
I have kept	the good fight.

All of these actions point to the dedication with which Paul pursued the prize of intimate fellowship with God. He had run to receive the crown of righteousness from the Lord.

- Who else did Paul say will receive this crown (v. 8)?

- What makes you feel that this group includes you?

Paul knew he would receive this crown by God's grace. Paul had already reminded Timothy of his absolute confidence in God's trustworthiness in 2 Timothy 1:12. You, like Paul, must learn to grow in confidence that God will guard what we have entrusted to Him.

In Philippians 1:9-11 Paul prayed that the believers would be filled with the fruit of righteousness that comes through Jesus Christ. Those who wear the crown of righteousness will produce the fruit of righteousness.

➳ Check the following words or phrases that would result from the fruit of righteousness:

- ☐ Abounding in love
- ☐ Awards
- ☐ Popularity
- ☐ Depth of insight
- ☐ Purity
- ☐ Blamelessness

In Revelation 4:4-11 the heavenly adoration and the crown of worship is described. Four living creatures and 24 elders gather around the throne of God and are consumed with the worship of God. Some scholars believe the 24 elders represent the whole Church that will praise and worship God in all His glory in heaven.

➳ What did the elders do with their crowns?

This is the greatest purpose of the crown. It is to be laid down as an act of worship before the One who created all things and is worthy of praise.

As you read Revelation 5:11-14, think about this picture and what it will be like to participate in uninterrupted praise to God with your whole being.

➳ Write a brief paragraph or draw a picture that expresses what you think it will be like to bow your knees and lift your voice to God in praise and worship on that day.

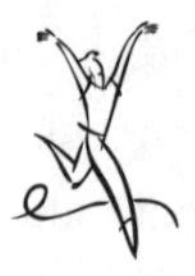

Father God, help me pursue Your righteousness and produce its fruit in my life.

Heavenly Father, I commit myself to You so that one day I can fall down and lay my crown before Your throne.

DAY 4: *The Crown of Love and Compassion*

The crown that God has for us includes love and compassion. In Psalm 103:1-4 David listed several actions for which he praised God.

From the following list, check three areas of your life in which you have experienced God's love and compassion the strongest during the last two years:

- ☐ Family
- ☐ Job
- ☐ Friends
- ☐ Health
- ☐ Church
- ☐ Finances

➳ Describe one of your blessings in one of these areas.

Love and compassion are sometimes translated as loving-kindness and tender mercies. The Old Testament prophets affirmed these attributes of God. In Isaiah 63:7-9 Isaiah described how God longs to bless us with His love and compassion for now and all eternity.

➳ Considering verse 9, tell about an incident in which you felt God lifted you up and carried you in His love.

In Psalms 21:1-3; 46:1 and 55:16-17, David tells us of God's love, mercy and compassion.

➳ After each Scripture reference, describe what God gives to those who trust in Him.

- Psalm 21:1-3

- Psalm 46:1

- Psalm 55:16-17

God's love came pouring out to us through Calvary, and Calvary's love leads to eternal salvation and a crown of love and compassion from the One who loves you most of all.

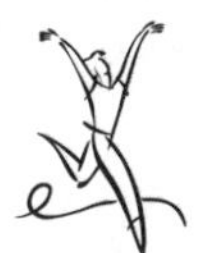

Father God, help me to pursue Your justice, righteousness and loving-kindness with all my heart and soul.

Father, I am unworthy of Your grace and mercy. Help me to worship You on bended knees with a contrite and humble heart.

DAY 5: *The Crown of Glory and Honor*

Another crown that we receive as a reward from God is described as a crown of glory and honor. This crown also appears as the crown of creation, coronation and celebration.

In Psalm 8:4-5, David praised God for bestowing on humans the crown of glory and honor. Sadly, many human beings do not claim their glory and honor that God created for them. Worldly systems do much to degrade and dehumanize. We sometimes dishonor our bodies by our lifestyles and habits.

➳ How has the First Place program helped you claim the crown of glory and honor that God bestowed on you at creation?

By emphasizing the stewardship of the body, mind and spirit, Christians can focus the world's attention on the glory and honor we have received from God through creation.

The crown of glory and honor has been worn by only a select few humans through the ages. Vashti and Esther, both queens of Persia, were two biblical women who wore crowns of glory and honor.

Esther 1:9-11 and Esther 2:15-18 describe the two queens.

- What is the difference between the two queens and their crowns?

- Why did Vashti lose her crown?

- Why did Esther receive her crown?

- What did Mordecai ask Esther to do in Esther 4:12-14 ?

- Think about your own family, job, church or First Place group. Has God put you where you are—for such a time as this? How do you know?

- What can you do today, tomorrow or this week to demonstrate God's purpose in your life?

- Which commitments have been the most helpful to you in your race for the prize?

- Think about any of the commitments that seem to be more difficult or take more of an effort to follow. What can you do to make these commitments easier to handle?

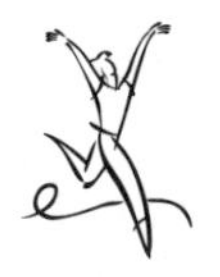

Father God, help me to follow the commitments of First Place.

Lord, give me the courage to accept Your crown of glory and honor and stand for You and help Your people in this world come to know You.

DAY 6: *Reflections*

What a wonderful message of hope is brought to you by this week's study. How can you help but praise and worship God as never before? The anticipation of standing before the throne of God and laying our crowns at His feet is a motivation like no other.

As you run the race for the prize, Scripture memorization, prayer and Bible study will draw you closer to the one true God. These spiritual weapons have divine power to enable you to overcome your strongholds and demolish them.

If you are still experiencing problems in memorizing Scripture, try something new. Along with the CD and book, develop a picture or association in your mind for each phrase or group of words. For example: Using the verse for this week, think of the first few words: "When the chief shepherd appears." You could mentally picture a shepherd leading his sheep. For "you will receive the crown of glory," picture the Olympic athletes getting a crown instead of a medal. "That will never fade away" brings to mind a parent's love that never dies. This verse is simple and not too difficult, but using this same technique for longer verses may help you picture the verse and remember it more quickly.

If you learn better by doing, then write the verse down several times a day and look at it. This helps you visualize the verse as you write each word. In addition, get into the habit of repeating the reference at the beginning and end of the verse. So many times people learn verses, then later can't recall where the Scripture is found.

Don't limit yourself to just memorizing the verse for the week. When you come across verses in the study that have special meaning to you, commit those verses to memory and use them as you pray.

Here are a few examples to help you get started:

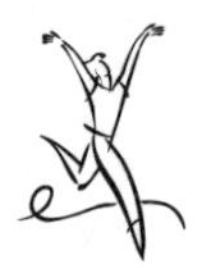

Lord, help me to resist temptation for I know the one who endures temptation will receive the crown of life that You have promised to those who love You (see James 1:12).

Father, I want to be able to say that I have fought the good fight, kept the faith and finished the race so that I may receive the crown of righteousness You have put aside for me on that day (see 2 Timothy 4:6-8).

Father God, thank You for abiding in me and letting me abide in You. You have promised that whatever I desire shall be done. Give me a right spirit so that my desires will be pleasing and bear much fruit for You (see John 15:7).

DAY 7: *Reflections*

During this week we have referred to the various crowns: crown of life, crown of glory and honor, crown of love and compassion, crown of rejoicing and crown of righteousness. The ultimate crown in all this is the crown of worship. Worship requires a right relationship with God and an understanding that His grace and mercy have been bestowed upon us.

The ultimate end with the crown of worship is not what you have done or how you have worshiped here but the glory of God Himself.

David knew what the worship of God meant. In Psalm 146:2 he wrote "I will praise the LORD all my life; I will sing praise to my God as long as I live." In Psalm 34:1 David told us to extol the Lord at all times. His praise should always be upon our lips.

Praise and worship of God come through prayer and Scripture. You may go to church for formal worship with fellow believers, but you can also worship every day as you read the Bible and pray. Memorize Scriptures that praise God and extol Him to the highest. You will find yourself drawing closer to Him each day.

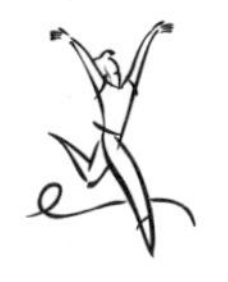

Dear Lord, let me continually offer to You a sacrifice of praise, the fruit of lips that confess Your name (see Hebrews 13:15).

Oh God, I bow down in worship; I kneel before You as my Lord, for You are my God and I am as the sheep of Your pasture (see Psalm 95:6-7).

Father God, I look forward to the day when the Chief Shepherd appears, and I will receive the crown of glory that will never fade away (see 1 Peter 5:4).

Group Prayer Requests Today's Date:_______________

Name	Request	Results

REMOVING EVERY OBSTACLE

Week Eight

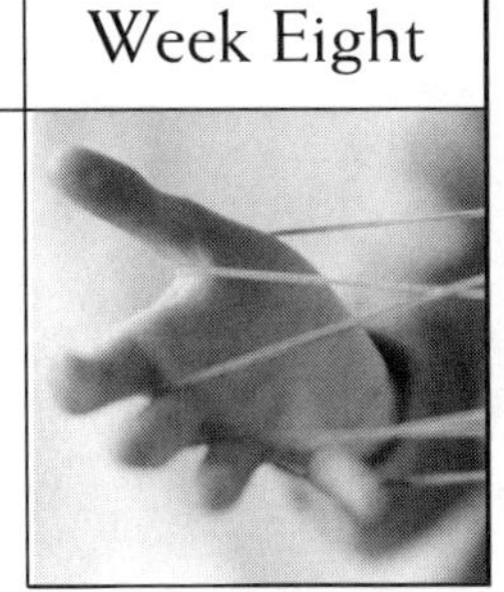

MEMORY VERSE

Therefore, since we are surrounded by such a great cloud of witnesses, let us throw off everything that hinders and the sin that so easily entangles, and let us run with perseverance the race marked out for us.

Hebrews 12:1

This week's study focuses on removing every obstacle as we press on to the prize. The memory verse reminds us that serious obstacles must be dealt with specifically. Otherwise, any or all of them can trip up the most skilled runner.

As you study this week, spend some extra time praying about those obstacles that trouble you most. The obstacles must not prevent you from pressing on!

DAY 1: *Loneliness*

Don't look now, but you're surrounded! This statement paraphrases the beginning of Hebrews 12. Loneliness is not simply being alone. It involves feelings of isolation and alienation even in the midst of a crowd. In Mark 3:31-35, although surrounded by a crowd of listeners and being sought by His family, Jesus expressed His realization that not everyone was with Him.

➳ Who did Jesus say were His true family?

One resource for dealing with loneliness is remembering the fact that God has surrounded us with those witnesses who have gone ahead of us as models—as described in Hebrews 11—and who cheer us on. Remembering those faithful ones can inspire you anew today.

- After reading Hebrews 11:32-40, list at least four of the actions of these heroes of faith.

- Name four of the hardships they endured.

Even as God provided encouragement and help for these heroes, He will put people in your life today to provide encouragement. Because everyone needs encouragement, First Place included it as one of the commitments. Your encouragement to someone else may provide just the motivation they need to press on.

- Name those from the past who serve to inspire you today. Your cloud of witnesses may be from the Bible or your own personal experience.

God promises never to leave us alone. He sent the Holy Spirit to comfort and encourage us. John 14:26-27 is the promise of that comforter.

- Describe a time in your life when you felt surrounded by God's love even though you were alone.

- List the persons in your life at the present time who inspire and encourage you.

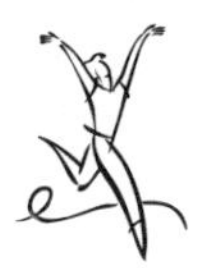

Father, give me Your power to lead me out of my dark wilderness. I know I am not alone, for You have surrounded me with many witnesses and the comfort of the Holy Spirit.

DAY 2: *Excessiveness and Restlessness*

The memory verse commands that we not be overwhelmed with excessiveness—having more activities on our plate than we could ever digest. Many times Christians become so involved with activities and service that we lose sight of the purpose of our service. We must learn to lay aside any encumbrance that would hinder or prevent us from pressing on.

In Luke 12:13-21 Jesus told a parable about someone who never had enough and was consumed with getting more. This problem could apply to religious and social activities as well as material gain.

- What was the rich man's desire?

- What happened to him?

- On a scale of 1 to 10, how productive for eternity do you see your life at the present time?

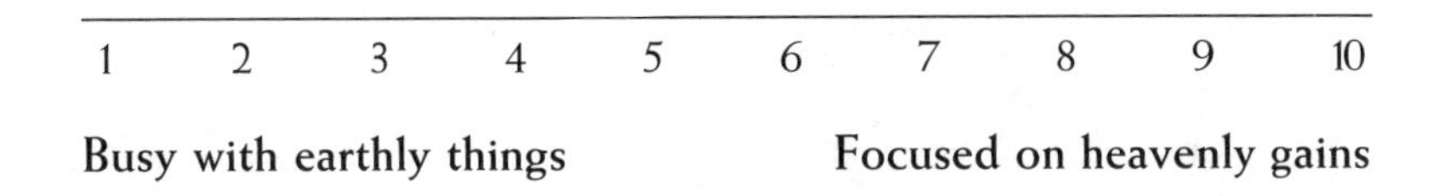

- When you are involved in too many things, what helps you narrow your focus and increase your sense of meaningful accomplishment?

Being caught up in excessiveness can also destroy effectiveness in your prayer life. You find yourself too busy to pray. God has given a model prayer to help us set our priorities.

➳ After reading Matthew 6:9-13, name the priorities found in this prayer.

When you are too busy in life doing service and activities, you may lose the patience to run with perseverance. You must learn to be patient in this restless world.

➳ After reading Revelation 14:6-7,12, mark T (for true) and F (for false) for the following statements concerning how believers are to accomplish patient endurance:

____ They must be busy day and night.
____ They must obey God's commandments.
____ They must remain faithful to Jesus.
____ They must read many books about patience.

In Matthew 11:28-30 Jesus gave us a very definite command about how to have patience and overcome restlessness.

➳ In what area has God given you rest from your impatience and restlessness?

➳ What area of restlessness do you need to surrender to God today?

Isaiah 40:28-31 gives us the encouragement to persevere and run the race with endurance. God promises strength and power when we trust and wait on Him.

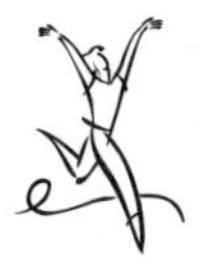

Oh Lord, I pray for Your will to be done in my life. Help me to remove excessiveness from my life.

Help me, Father God, to wait on You in such a way so that I will run and not be tired. Lighten every step of my way.

DAY 3: *Possessiveness and Nosiness*

Possessiveness is the desire to have as much as a person can grab and hold on to. The obstacle of possessiveness hinders our spiritual development. It leads us to the false conclusion that we can't trust God to care for us. Christian stewardship removes the weight of possessiveness. Stewardship recognizes God's ownership of all things. He calls on us to manage His creation and the things He has given us as His stewards.

Stewardship begins with the management of ourselves and our bodies.

➳ Complete the following sentences:

- Your body is a ________________________________.
- You were bought ________________________________.
- Therefore, honor ________________________________.

➳ How has First Place helped you to develop good stewardship of God's temple—your body?

We must also be good stewards of our relationships with others. In 1 Samuel 1:21-28 Hannah demonstrated godly stewardship by committing her son Samuel to God.

➳ Give an example of how you have let go of the control of someone you love and given him or her to God. Or tell how you can be less possessive toward a specific person.

One obstacle that may hurt relationships with others is nosiness. The memory verse reminds us to run the race marked out for us. If we give all our energy toward running our own race, we won't have time or energy to meddle in the spiritual or personal concerns of others.

In 2 Thessalonians 3:10-13 and 1 Timothy 5:13, Paul warned the believers about the problem of nosiness related to idleness.

- Why does idleness often lead to being nosy about others' personal lives?

- How can we avoid meddling in others' lives?

In 1 Peter 4:12-17 Peter encouraged believers to praise God for being able to suffer for His name. He used the word "meddler" to describe a busybody. Peter says you are not to be such a person if you want to be a good witness to non-Christians.

- What can you do as a Christian to keep your care and concern about another person from turning into nosiness?

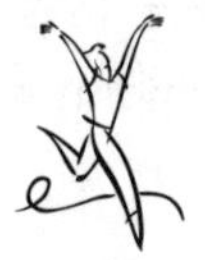

Father God, help me pursue with endurance the race You have set for me. Help me to let go of my wrong priorities and focus only on You.

Lord God, help me to keep my nose in place as a testimony to my claiming Your grace.

Day 4: *Worldliness*

Worldliness hinders us as we press on to the prize of intimate fellowship with God. This perspective loses sight of eternal values as it focuses on the prizes and pleasures of the moment. No one struggled any more with this obstacle than Samson, a judge of Israel.

➳ After reading Judges 14:1-7,19-20;16:1-6, check the words in the following list that describe Samson's problems with worldliness:

- ☐ Selfishness
- ☐ Greed
- ☐ Vandalism
- ☐ Immorality
- ☐ Murder
- ☐ Rebellion

Do you see that *all* of the words accurately represent Samson? Although he finally demonstrated faith in God to defeat his enemies, his worldliness brought misery on himself and others.

➳ Do any of the words listed in the previous activity describe an area of worldliness that has been particularly difficult for you? If so, how have you tried to overcome this stronghold?

➳ In Titus 2:11-14 Paul encouraged believers in Christ to claim God's grace to overcome worldliness. Match the following phrases to correctly complete Paul's instructions:

____ We must say no to	a. godly lives in the present age.
____ We must live	b. eager to do good.
____ We must wait	c. worldly passions.
____ We must be	d. for Christ's return.

➳ Which of these instructions do you need to implement? Why?

In Romans 12:1-2 Paul points out that a transformed mind can help produce a life not conformed to a worldly perspective.

- How have you seen God use the First Place program to transform your mind and body from worldliness to godliness?

Worldliness is such a heavy weight to carry when running the race of the Christian life. It caused even a very strong man like Samson to be defeated. But we can remove this stronghold if we determine to have our minds daily renewed by God's grace.

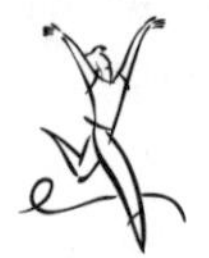

Father God, help me to use my First Place group and other Christian friends to give me the support I need to overcome the worldly perspectives that are all around me.

DAY 5: *Pride*

Hebrews 12:1 counsels you to throw off the sin that so easily entangles. It pictures an item of clothing that wraps itself around a runner's legs, causing him to stumble and fall. One obstacle or spiritual stronghold that entangles your life, trying to trip you up, is pride.

In the Bible, pride is described as arrogance of heart and mind that causes us to seek only our own best interest. Pride is an incumbrance that must be laid aside.

- What does Proverbs 16:18-19 tell you about pride?

- What characteristic should we seek instead?

Two men in the Old Testament dealt with their pride in diverse ways with different outcomes. First, Hezekiah, king of Judah, offended God with his proud heart.

- After reading 2 Chronicles 32:22-26, place a check by the thing that angered God the most about Hezekiah's pride.

  - ☐ He was unwilling to ask for God's help.
  - ☐ He was uncaring about his nation.
  - ☐ He was unresponsive to God's kindness.
  - ☐ He was unconcerned about his enemies.

After Hezekiah stirred up God's wrath, he finally repented of his pride, and God withheld His wrath. King Belshazzar of Babylon is the second example of one who held on to his pride.

- After reading Daniel 5:17-23, check the accusations Daniel made against the king about his pride.

  - ☐ He failed to humble himself.
  - ☐ He failed to learn from his father.
  - ☐ He worshiped idols and not God.
  - ☐ He honored Daniel with an exalted position.

Pride comes from doing things our own way and not being responsive to God and others.

- What is an area of pride in your life?

- According to 1 John 2:16-17, what happens to pride (boasting of what one has and does)?

➳ What is the reward for one who does the will of God?

You are not to love the world or things in the world, but your purpose is to do the will of God. Then you will reap the reward of the prize for which God calls you heavenward.

➳ What do you need to do to surrender your pride and humble yourself before God?

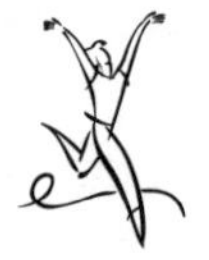

Father God, help me to seek after You and lay aside pride. Give me wisdom and humility as I forsake worldly things and seek Your will.

Lord, give me the courage to lay aside everything that entangles me and keeps me from running the race You marked for me.

DAY 6: *Reflections*

This week's study has shown us a number of obstacles that can quickly become strongholds in our lives. Loneliness, excessiveness, possessiveness, nosiness, worldliness, pride and restlessness can come into our lives and push out those things that can help us run with endurance and perseverance.

Strongholds take over and consume the time and energy you need to focus on the goal of true intimate fellowship with God. Confessing these sins and seeking forgiveness can help to get you back on course. When you are seeking God and His will, you don't have time for the obstacles that can hinder your race. When God's Word fills your time, the sins that entangle have a difficult time getting a stronghold. The more Scriptures you have committed to memory, the more power you have against the things of the world.

Don't limit yourself to just memorizing the verse for the week. When you come across verses in the study that have special meaning to you, commit those verses to memory and use them as you pray. Repeat the verse often each day, and then use it each day in conversation or in prayer to help you remember it.

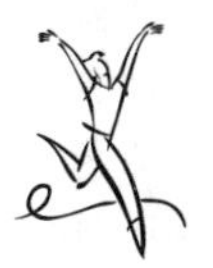

Lord, help me to overcome loneliness. You have promised to not leave me comfortless or alone. You have sent the Holy Spirit to comfort and guide me (see John 14:16,18).

God, thank You for disciplining me for my good, that I may share in Your holiness (see Hebrews 12:10).

You have shown me what is good. And what do You, Lord, require of me? To act justly and to love mercy and to walk humbly with You, my God (see Micah 6:8).

DAY 7: *Reflections*

When strongholds take over your life and begin to choke out the Word, it is time to go deeper into the Scriptures and find God's answers for you. Only God can help you overcome any of the strongholds discussed this week. Each one can enter your life in such subtle ways that you may not be aware of it until you find it taking over your time and thoughts.

Scripture memory may be the obstacle that is keeping you from being in complete fellowship with God because you believe memorization is too hard for you. Now is the time to press on with perseverance and trust God to help you. Use the CD and the Scripture memory book as aids in memorizing your verses each week. In addition, study the verse in context and try to understand what it means.

Memorizing Scripture takes a commitment of your time and a willing heart. Develop a positive attitude and say with Paul, "I can do everything through him who gives me strength" (Philippians 4:13).

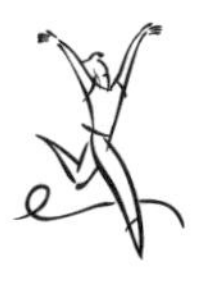

Father, You are teaching me that pride only breeds quarrels, but wisdom is found in those who take advice. Help me to discern when pride is involved in my quarrels (see Proverbs 13:10).

My faithful Father, You've warned me that when pride comes, then comes disgrace, but with humility comes wisdom (see Proverbs 11:2).

Lord God, You have told me that my body is a temple of the Holy Spirit and I was bought at a great price. Help me to honor You with my body and to live a life worthy of Your calling (see 1 Corinthians 6:19-20).

Heavenly Father, You have surrounded me with a great cloud of witnesses. Let me get rid of everything that hinders me and the sin that entangles me so that I may run with perseverance the race You have marked out for me (see Hebrews 12:1).

Group Prayer Requests Today's Date:_______________

Name	Request	Results

LOOKING TO JESUS

Week Nine

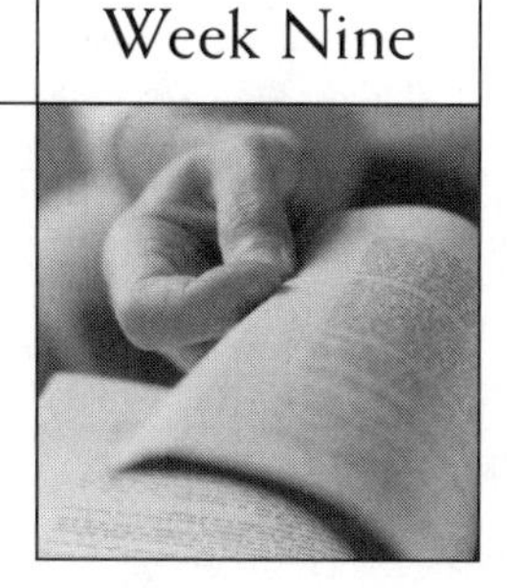

MEMORY VERSE

Let us fix our eyes on Jesus, the author and perfecter of our faith, who for the joy set before him endured the cross, scorning its shame, and sat down at the right hand of the throne of God.

Hebrews 12:2

The memory verse for this week encourages us to go beyond removing every obstacle to focusing on Jesus.

Surely nothing stimulates the believer to press on more than recognizing that Jesus has gone before us and goes with us now as we run the race set for us. God knows what is ahead for each of us; He has prepared the way, and He has prepared us for what lies ahead. John 12:20-21 relates the story of some Greeks who approached the disciples and with boldness told Philip, "We would like to see Jesus." In this week's study, we will look at seven biblical pictures of Jesus.

DAY 1: *Miracle Worker*

Let's begin with a fresh glimpse of Jesus as the miracle worker. A miracle is an event with a supernatural cause. The explanation for a real miracle is that only God could have done it. Jesus' miracles are evidence that God sent Him.

➳ Read John 10:36-38. Check the statement that Jesus gave as the reason to believe that He is God's Son.

- ☐ His disciples said it.
- ☐ His parables taught it.
- ☐ His miracles proved it.

After reading John 9:1-7, match the phrases that demonstrate what Jesus wanted His disciples to learn from this miracle.

____	God's work would be displayed	a. to be the world's light.
____	Jesus had to do the work	b. in the blind man's life.
____	Jesus was in the world	c. of the One who sent Him.

Jesus wanted His disciples to know that miracles come from God, meeting human needs in a supernatural way to display His glory.

Many people may wonder, *Do miracles still occur today?* In John 14:10-14, Jesus affirmed that His followers would do greater things than He did.

➳ Why would Jesus state that?

➳ After reading John 14:10-14, complete the statement that explains the purpose of miracles today.

And I will do whatever you ________________________ in my name, so that the ________________________________ may bring glory to the ____________________________________.

Miracles today include healing of body, mind, emotions, finances and relationships, but we also experience miracles in everyday ways that we may not readily recognize. The miracles that occur today are God's handiwork through the Holy Spirit working in the lives of those who love Him.

The miracles of Jesus brought joy to the hearts and lives of those whom He touched. Mary and Martha rejoiced when Jesus restored the life of their brother, Lazarus. One healed leper came to Jesus to thank Him for healing the leprosy and giving him new life. Christians today need to reflect the joy that Jesus gives.

➳ What miracle do you need to thank God for?

- In Philippians 4:4, what action did Paul twice state that we must do?

- How can you rejoice even in times of difficulty?

If you rejoice in praise and thanksgiving, you will be blessed. When you cast your cares on Him, surrender that heavy burden and let Him carry the load, He will restore His joy to you. (See Matthew 11:29-30; Psalm 30:10-12.)

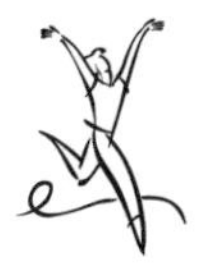

Heavenly Father, display Your power and love for me through the miracles You perform in my life and the lives of others.

Lord God, give me victory over my burdens and let me cast all my cares on You. Restore to me the joy that only You can give.

DAY 2: *Kingdom Teacher*

The Gospels portray Jesus not only as a miracle worker but also as the Kingdom teacher.

- According to Mark 1:14-18, what was Jesus' message about the kingdom of God?

The kingdom of God is the rule of God in our lives. Believers are to follow Jesus in every area of their lives. Jesus' kingdom is the kingdom of God and of heaven, not of men and of Earth.

Jesus taught about the kingdom of God through parables. A parable is an earthly story with a heavenly meaning. He used parables so that His disciples would understand the principles He wanted them to know. He consistently taught that the kingdom of God is unlike any earthly kingdom.

In Mark 4:30-34 Jesus compared God's kingdom to the mustard seed.

- In your own words write the parable of the mustard seed.

- How has the kingdom of God grown like the mustard seed in your life?

In Matthew 13:44-46 Jesus pointed out that the kingdom of God is more valuable than any earthly kingdom. Compare the two parables in the following chart to discover the common thread in both:

	Parable 1 (v. 44)	Parable 2 (vv. 45-46)
What was found		
Action taken		

- How has the value of the kingdom of God grown in your understanding?

- What part has your participation in First Place had in that growth?

Jesus valued His role as the Kingdom teacher. Everything He said and did conformed to His heart's desire for you to understand and enter the kingdom of God.

According to Mark 10:13-15, Jesus taught that the kingdom of God belongs to the children, and that you must have childlike faith to enter the Kingdom.

➳ Briefly explain what Jesus meant when He said we must be like a child to enter His kingdom.

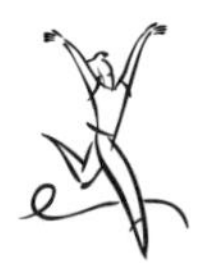

Lord, give me the faith of a child that I too may enter the kingdom of God.

Father, help me to live worthy of Your kingdom.

DAY 3: *Faith Author*

We have looked at portraits of Jesus as the miracle worker and the Kingdom teacher. Let's look at the images of Jesus as found in this week's memory verse. The first is that Jesus is the author of our faith. Faith originates with Jesus Christ, the Alpha and the Omega, the beginning and the ending (see Revelation 1:8).

➳ What does John 1:1-8 tell us about Jesus?

The Bible is the written Word of God that points sinners to the living Word of God. The Bible teaches us the lifestyle that honors Christ. However, the Bible does not save us. Salvation is found only by faith in Jesus Christ.

After reading 2 Timothy 3:16-17, put a check by the following words that indicate what the Bible is useful for:

☐ Teach	☐ Equip
☐ Reconcile	☐ Fulfill
☐ Forgive	☐ Cleanse
☐ Correct	☐ Train

The Bible is there for teaching, but it teaches that only Jesus, the living Word of God, is able to forgive, reconcile, cleanse and fulfill sinners.

➳ How did God use the Bible to confront you with your need to put your trust in Christ?

Scripture memory will help you overcome obstacles that may keep you from pressing on. Just as the Scriptures led you to your faith in Christ, they will teach you and guide you into the right way of living and serving God.

Remember the story of Abraham, as briefly described in Hebrews 11:8? Abraham obeyed when God called him, even though he didn't know where he was going.

➳ Describe a time when you stepped out on faith even though you were not sure where it would lead you. What were the results?

➳ What do Matthew 21:21-22 and Mark 11:22-24 tell you about your faith in Jesus?

➳ What do John 2:11 and 11:45 tell you about faith?

Hebrews 11 is a roll call of the heroes of faith of the Old Testament—men and women who stepped out in faith to obey God. The faith that God gives you today was the same faith that these heroes of old had. They set the example, and their testimonies give inspiration and courage to Christians today.

Jesus Christ is the author of your faith too. Don't keep it hidden within yourself. Look for an opportunity to share your salvation experience with someone who does not know Christ. Encourage someone with the idea that God's blessings are abundant and His promises sure. Just sharing what Christ means to you and what He has done for you will be a blessing to both of you!

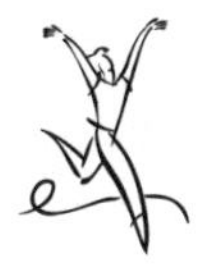

Father God, give me the courage to step out on faith and trust everything I have to You, for You promised to answer my prayers when I pray in faith, believing in You.

Lord God, thank You for sending Your Son to bear my sins on the cross. Give me the boldness to witness to others and tell them what You have done in my life and will do for them.

DAY 4: *Faith Perfecter and Eternal Ruler*

Jesus is the perfecter of our faith. He gives us the Holy Spirit for "attaining to the whole measure of the fullness of Christ" (Ephesians 4:13). Unlike Christ, none of us are capable of living sinless lives. However, we can become dedicated to doing God's will.

➳ In Philippians 1:6, Paul describes the confidence he had in God. Write in your own words what Paul had learned.

➳ How can you cooperate with God in completing His work in you?

➳ After reading Hebrews 4:14-16, complete the following statements. We can have confidence in Christ to perfect our faith because:

He is able to sympathize with our ________________________.

He was tempted in ________________________ just as we are.

He will give us grace in our time of ________________________.

God is also our eternal ruler. He sits on the throne to show His preeminence in all things. Jesus has the highest place of honor, sitting on the Father's right side.

In much of the book of Revelation, God the Father is pictured as sitting on a throne. Jesus is also pictured as the exalted Lord, sitting on His throne.

➳ Revelation 3:21 contains great promises. Complete the following statement:

To him who ________________, I will give the right to sit with ________________ on my ________________, just as I overcame and ________________ down with my ________________ on his throne.

Jesus claimed His own throne while still maintaining the difference between His and His Father's thrones. However, the great promise is that His followers who overcome Satan's attacks will sit with Him on His throne. Jesus is preparing to share His throne with you!

➳ What do you overcome in your life in view of the fact that you will someday reign with Christ?

Many believers happily begin in faith but sadly have not matured in faith. Many have seen Jesus hanging on the cross or rising from the empty tomb. They may not see Him seated on His throne at the Father's right hand in glory and power and not see themselves seated with Jesus on His throne. Having confidence in Christ to perfect your faith allows Him to mature you so that you can claim your privileges as a child of the King and someday reign with Him.

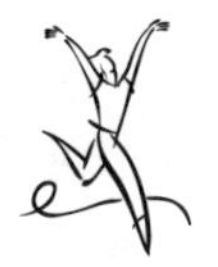

Lord God, give me confidence to approach Your throne of grace so that I may receive mercy and find grace to help me in my time of need.

Heavenly Father, help me to live up to the position and privilege I have as a child of the King.

DAY 5: *Cross and Shame Bearer*

Hebrews 12:2 specifies that only Jesus could win our salvation. Jesus was the cross bearer for all sinners and thus became our Savior.

Isaiah 53:3-6 helps us to understand all that Jesus did to bear our sins.

- What are your feelings as you read Isaiah 53:3-6?

- Colossians 2:13-15 describes what God did for us through the cross. Check the following statements that tell you what God did when Jesus bore the cross:

  - ☐ God gave us eternal life.
  - ☐ He forgave us all our sins.
  - ☐ He canceled our debt to the law.
  - ☐ He disarmed the powers of evil.
  - ☐ He set us free from religious rule keeping.

Because Jesus is our cross bearer, we do not have to earn our own salvation, and in fact we can check all five statements.

- Write a paragraph or draw a picture describing Jesus' actions on your behalf. Think of Him as your cross bearer; then express your feelings.

The second part of the memory verse states that Jesus endured the cross and scorned its shame "for the joy set before him." He endured the cross because He knew it completely defeated sin. In the midst of the shame and tragedy, His joy came from God and from fulfilling His purpose.

Hebrews 12:2 makes it clear that, although the cross was not a happy experience for Jesus, His joy overflowed because of His overwhelming victory over sin. Jesus chose not to focus on the shame of bearing the cross, but on the joyful result—our salvation from sin!

Consider Matthew 27:27-31. The shame Jesus endured from the soldiers alone was enough to crush the will of most men, but Jesus bore the shame for you and me.

- List at least three examples of the shame Jesus had to endure from people.

- Have you felt shamed by people? Describe the experience.

Can you imagine how much greater our perfect Savior's shame must have been in comparison to the shame you felt in the experience you just described?

Father God, I look at the Cross and cannot begin to comprehend such love that would bear the shame and ridicule of the people. Help me, O Mighty God, to live each day in praise and honor of such a great sacrifice.

Lord, thank You for setting me free to live a holy, upright life guided by Your teachings. I love You, Jesus, my cross bearer.

DAY 6: *Reflections*

This week's study has shown us how Jesus is our cross bearer. He paid the price for sin that no one else could pay. While being that cross bearer, He claimed the joy of total victory over sin rather than submitting to the defeat of great shame. If He could scorn the shame of everyone's sin, surely He can give you victory over your sin.

The strongholds of sin will become heavy burdens. When Christians allow anything but God to be exalted in their minds, their focus is lost and they will feel overpowered. Has this happened to you? Whether the stronghold is an addiction, unforgiveness, despair over a loss or rebellion, it consumes so much of your emotional and mental energy that your abundant life is strangled. Memorizing Scriptures and praying give Satan a difficult time in getting a foothold in your life. The more Scriptures you have committed to memory, the more power you have against the things of the world.

Jesus wants to continue to bear your burdens. Review Matthew 11:28-30. Yes, He has promised to give you rest for your weary soul. Take up your cross and you will find that He carries the heavy load for you. You will have victory in Jesus and a blessed assurance that Jesus is your Savior. You belong to Him.

The Word of God is your weapon against the world. Read it daily, listen to its message, commit the words to memory; then use them wisely in your struggles against the temptations that distract you from your goal to win the prize.

Lord, help me to persevere under trial, for You have said that when I stand the test, I will receive the crown of life that You promise to those who love You (see James 1:12).

Father God, as the perfecter and author of my faith, help me to walk by that faith and not by sight (see 2 Corinthians 5:7).

Heavenly Father, let me hold on to my shield of faith so that I can quench all the fiery darts hurled at me by the world and the wicked one (see Ephesians 6:16).

DAY 7: *Reflections*

Many times Christians picture Jesus hanging on the cross or rising from the empty tomb. Artists through the centuries have depicted these scenes on canvas and in sculpture. However, many do not picture Him on the throne at the Father's right hand in glory and power. As a child of the King, you will someday reign with Him. Claim your privilege as a child of the King in your everyday living. Claim Revelation 3:20-21 as your birthright into the kingdom of God.

Scripture memory becomes the tool by which you let others see Jesus reigning in your life. You can become an encouragement to others who are having difficult times. Living in close relationship to Him will give you the incentive and motivation you need to exercise your body and nourish it. By doing these things, you will bring honor and glory to God through your witness and example.

You have the weapons of prayer and God's Word to become strong and powerful against all foes. Pick up your weapons each day and prepare to do battle with the devil, who is prowling around like a roaring lion, just waiting for someone he can devour. The roaring lion will back down and slink away when confronted by the power of God through Scripture and prayer.

Kneel down, come to the throne of grace and be filled with the love and grace of God. Claim your position, focus on the prize and run the race marked out for you.

Lord Jesus, You stood at the door of my heart and knocked. I let You in and You dined with me. Help me to continue to hear Your knock and let You in. I look forward to the day when I will sit with You on the throne just as You sat down with Your Father on His throne (see Revelation 3:20-21).

My faithful Father, I have sinned and like a sheep gone astray; I have turned to my own desires and ways. I seek Your forgiveness, for You were oppressed and afflicted in silence and led like a lamb to the slaughter to bear my shame and guilt. All my sins were laid on You (see Isaiah 53:6-7).

Holy God, I do not want to grieve Your Holy Spirit by whom I was sealed for the day of redemption. Take away all bitterness, wrath, anger, clamor and evil speaking, and help me be kind to others. Give me a tender heart and a willingness to forgive others even as You have forgiven me through Christ (see Ephesians 4:30-32).

Lord Jesus, I focus on You, the author and perfecter of my faith. You endured the cross, scorned its shame and sat down at the right hand of the throne of God. Thank You for loving me (see Hebrews 12:2).

GROUP PRAYER REQUESTS TODAY'S DATE:______________

NAME	REQUEST	RESULTS

GOD'S LOVE FOR YOU

Week Ten

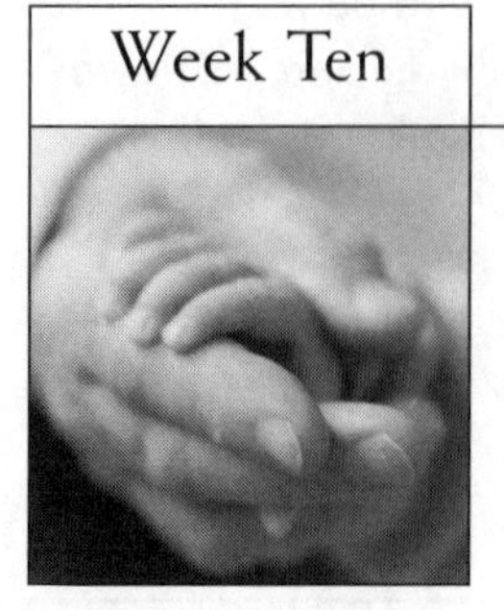

MEMORY VERSE

See to it that no one misses the grace of God
and that no bitter root grows up
to cause trouble and defile many.
Hebrews 12:15

As children we were taught that some things are poisonous. We were warned, "Don't drink that. It might kill you!" Many children are alive today because they took that warning seriously.

The memory verse for this week is a warning about something that could poison us. Hebrews 12:15 warns us that we should not miss the grace of God. Then we are warned not to let a poisonous bitter root grow within us. This week's study shows us seven avenues for accepting God's grace. Surely nothing is more important in pressing on to the prize than focusing on God's grace.

DAY 1: *Becoming a Grace-Filled Believer*

Hebrews 12:15 begins with the warning, "See to it that no one misses the grace of God." Grace means unmerited favor. Grace is God's blessing that we cannot earn from anything we do. So how do we become grace-filled believers?

- What is Paul's description of grace in Ephesians 2:8-9?

- Choose two aspects of this description and explain how God has specifically demonstrated these truths to you.

- In light of these truths about grace, write in your own words why Hebrews 12:15 insists that God's grace must not be missed by any believer.

- Since grace cannot be earned or deserved, you must put aside your pride to receive it. What areas of pride have you had to give up in order to receive God's grace through faith?

Becoming a grace-filled believer requires that you move beyond any claims of goodness for yourself. There is nothing of yourself that you can boast about. There is nothing that you need that you do not receive from His grace.

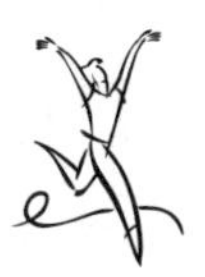

Dear Lord, help me to bask in Your grace and the all-sufficient supply You have for me.

Heavenly Father, help me to grow in the grace and knowledge of my Lord and Savior Jesus Christ.

DAY 2: *Living Peaceably and Practicing Forgiveness*

Hebrews 12:14 commands, "Make every effort to live in peace with all men." Is such a command possible to fulfill?

In Colossians 3:12-15 there are five reasons why believers must let the peace of Christ rule in their hearts.

- Complete each reason for letting the peace of Christ rule in your heart.

1. You are God's chosen ________________.
2. You are dearly ________________.
3. The Lord forgave ________________.
4. You are members of one ________________.
5. You were called to ________________.

- According to Ephesians 4:30-31, what traits must we get rid of in order not to grieve the Holy Spirit?

- Which of these traits do you most desire to eliminate?

If you have an unforgiving heart toward anyone, your peace will be shattered. To maintain peace, you must continually forgive those who hurt you and ask forgiveness of those you have hurt. Recognizing this as a constant need can go a long way toward giving you peace and helping you to experience the grace of God.

Genesis 25:27-34 tells the story of twin brothers, Jacob and Esau, who were at odds with one another.

- What did Esau do to satisfy his hunger?

Later Jacob went even further by deceiving his father and stealing Esau's blessing too. Genesis 27:15-29 tells of that deception. If anyone needed forgiveness for what he did, Jacob did.

- What evidence do we see in Genesis 33:8-17 that Esau forgave his brother Jacob?

- Write the name of a person with whom you need to open lines of communication and make peace; then write a way to make peace with him or her.

- Have you forgiven a great hurt from someone else? How were you able to demonstrate forgiveness to that person?

Forgiveness must be understood as a process that has to be carefully pursued.

- In Mark 11:25-26 what was Jesus' command and what happens if you don't forgive?

- Review the Scriptures for today's study. What have you learned about having peace through a forgiving spirit?

- How will you apply it to your own life so that you do not miss the grace of God?

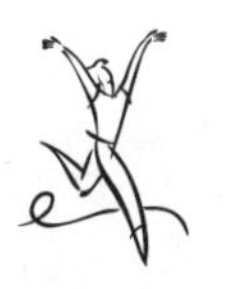

Lord, teach me to forgive others when they hurt me so that I may be forgiven my sins and trespasses.

Father, help me to be at peace with my enemies and not to judge others lest I be in danger of Your judgment.

DAY 3: *Seeking Holiness and Claiming an Unshakable Kingdom*

Focusing on God's grace leads believers to seek holiness. Without developing holiness we will miss seeing God at work. Hebrews 12:14 tells us to live in peace with all men and to be holy.

- Why do Christians need to make peace even with non-Christians ("all men") and be holy?

- According to Leviticus 20:26, why are we to be holy?

The word "consecrated" describes what is meant by holiness. It means being set apart, dedicated, devoted irrevocably to the worship of God with our lives.

- Read Exodus 19:6 in which God is preparing to give Moses the Ten Commandments. Before giving the commandments to His people in chapter 20, what did God tell them He was doing?

Read 1 Peter 2:9-12. Just as Israel was God's holy nation, Christians today are His holy people.

- What are the four titles given to Christians in verse 9?

God has set you apart as one of His chosen people. This should make a difference in the way you live.

- Identify one difference this should make in each of the following ways:

  - The way you take care of your body ____________________

    ____

  - Your attitude toward sin ____________________________

    ____

  - Your willingness to serve the Lord ____________________

    ____

To be holy and chosen means we can claim an unshakable Kingdom for our eternal home. The kingdom of God is the rule of God, and citizens of this kingdom are under the authority, power and protection of our heavenly King. The fact that this is an unshakable Kingdom undergirds us as believers. In Hebrews Paul encouraged us to gain strength for the race by meditating on the Kingdom that endures forever.

- Read the good news in Hebrews 12:28 and explain it in your own words.

In His testimony before Pilate in John 18:33-38, Jesus made some important claims about this unshakable Kingdom.

- What did Jesus mean when He said that His kingdom is not of this world?

- What difference does it make in your life to be part of the Kingdom that cannot be shaken or destroyed?

- What are you learning and experiencing in the First Place program that can help you live as a citizen of God's unshakable kingdom?

In both the Old and New Testaments, God challenged His people to be holy, just as He is holy. They are to be set apart and to live lives of holiness. The reward is a place in the unshakable kingdom of God.

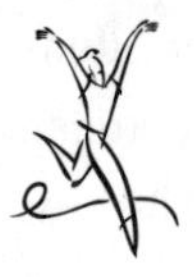

Heavenly Father, give me the courage to be completely set apart for Your glory.

Lord God, help me to live in such a way that Your rule will be evident in my life.

DAY 4: *Fleeing Immorality*

On Day 2 you learned about Esau selling his birthright to his brother Jacob for food. Hebrews 12:16 explains that Esau was a godless man willing to sell his inheritance for a single meal.

Genesis 25:29-34 describes the circumstances that led Esau to do something foolish that he would later regret.

- What were the three conditions that led Esau to do what he later regretted?

- Have you attempted to satisfy a physical need in the wrong way?

- Write a prayer of confession about this incident and seek God's forgiveness.

- Do you recall a time when you exchanged a future blessing for the momentary pleasure of food? How has God been working in your life to deliver you from this temptation?

After making his tragic mistake, Esau was in need of the grace of God. Unfortunately, Esau resisted God's grace. He allowed the root of bitterness to grow in place of grace.

- Read Genesis 28:6-9. Check the following statement that might indicate why Esau married a Canaanite woman:

  - ☐ He wanted to get back at his brother Jacob.
  - ☐ He wanted to hurt his father and mother.
  - ☐ He couldn't find anyone else to marry him.

2 Samuel 11:1-5 is another example of how immorality displeases God.

- What caused David to sin?

- According to 2 Samuel 12:9-14, what were the consequences of David's immorality?

- Have you ever been tempted to do something that was entirely out of God's will? How did you deal with the situation? What were the consequences?

Read Psalm 51:1-4,10-13, in which David repented from his sin and sought the mercy of God.

- What do these verses mean to you as you seek to repent and seek God's mercy in helping you flee from immorality?

Esau's life illustrates the truth of the memory verse that warns the more the root of bitterness takes hold in our hearts, the more it "grows up to cause trouble and defile many." David's life illustrates the truth that true repentance can bring forgiveness and blessing. Esau blamed others—David took all the blame on himself.

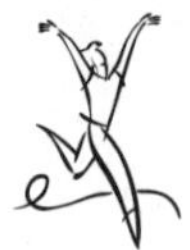

Lord God, keep me from blaming others for my mistakes. Help me to accept responsibility when I go astray.

Heavenly Father, Your Word says that as Your child, I was called to be free. Please help me not to use my freedom to indulge the sinful nature; rather help me to use my freedom to serve others in love.

DAY 5: *Expressing Thankfulness*

Expressing thankfulness on a regular basis assures a continuous focus on God's grace.

- According to Hebrews 12:28, how are we to worship God?

Thankfulness leads to the true worship of God. Such worship stems from the heart's desire to praise God. Both the Old and New Testaments instruct believers to praise God.

Throughout the psalms you will notice songs of praise and thanksgiving. The Psalms from 146 to 150 begin and end with the phrase "Praise the LORD."

- According to Psalm 148, none of God's creatures are excluded from praising Him! List the beings and things that are commanded to praise God.

Praising God and giving thanks is not something that comes naturally to most people. Sometimes praise seems more like lip service or something to be done at the beginning of prayer before getting to the wants and needs or supplications. However, the psalmist David wrote praises and thanksgiving to God that tell you to praise God wherever you are, at all times and for all things because God is worthy of your praise.

In the acronym ACTS used to guide prayer, *adoration* is the first thing to do in prayer. After *confessing* sin, you are to give *thanks* to God for what He has done for you before *asking* (supplication) Him for anything. Many churches sing the "Doxology" as a regular part of their worship services. The first line says, "Praise God from whom all blessings flow." When you think of the blessings you have as a child of the King, how can you help but praise and give thanks?

As you read Revelation 19:1-10, consider what an experience it will be to shout "Hallelujah! For our Lord God Almighty reigns!" One reason for our rejoicing is the privilege of participating in the wedding supper of the Lamb. Of particular interest are the words of the angel to John.

➳ What is the angel's command found in verse 10?

Expressing thankfulness is one of the highest forms of worshiping God. In your prayer journal list some things for which you are most thankful. Make it a habit to list each day three things for which you are thankful.

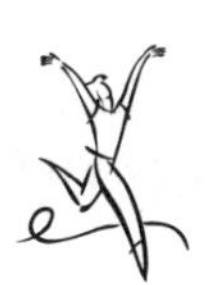

Father God, let my voice ring out in praises and thanksgiving to You for all the sacrifices You made for me and the blessings You have given me.

Lord Jesus, I praise You with a thankful heart. Thank You for Your constant love and care, and help me to press on in my devotion and service to You.

Day 6: *Reflections*

This week's study has revealed how much God loves each of us. He has filled us with grace, given us peace and forgiveness and promised an unshakable Kingdom where we can live forever with Him.

One of the conditions of claiming that Kingdom is to confess sin and flee immorality. Just as David turned from his immorality with Bathsheba, so we must turn from any sin that separates us from God and His blessing.

Throughout this study you have been taught how to overcome those strongholds by praising and worshiping God in prayer and Scripture. Prayer and God's Word are the most powerful weapons on Earth with which to defeat Satan. Beth Moore refers to them as sticks of dynamite bound together, and ignited with faith in what God says He can do.[1]

In the process of demolishing strongholds, the objective is to cast down anything that exalts itself in thought and take that thought captive for Christ. Do not allow anything or anyone to be exalted in your mind but Christ! You've learned to memorize Scripture and how to pray using Scripture during this study. These are tools and concepts that are used throughout the First Place Bible studies. Prayer keeps you in constant communion with God, which is necessary to press on to the prize for which God has called you. Prayer is the path to personal intimacy with Him that produces abundant living.

Review all the Bible verses you have memorized during this session and make each one a prayer to keep you focused on the ultimate prize of fellowship with your Lord and Savior.

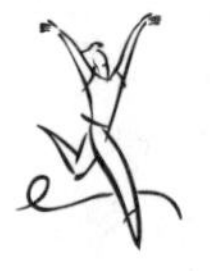

Father, Your Word exhorts me to set my mind on things above, not on earthly things. This can be such a battle, Lord! Please help me every single day to set my mind on You (see Colossians 3:2).

Father God, I ask You to lead me when I'm blinded by ways I do not know—along unfamiliar paths please guide me. Lord, turn the darkness into light before me and make the rough places smooth. These are the things You will do; I know You will not forsake me (see Isaiah 42:16).

DAY 7: *Reflections*

Praise and thanksgiving are other weapons against Satan. When the praise comes from God's Word and is combined with prayers of thanksgiving, you have a formidable force to protect you from the temptations of Satan.

When you worship God with praise and thanksgiving, you are showing the demons of darkness that your great God is worthy of praise.

God is worthy of your praise no matter what the circumstances. Praise is the shortcut to victory. In an earlier lesson (p. 46) praise was compared to the icons on a computer that offer shortcuts to programs and applications. Praise brings victory and victory evokes praise. It is a cycle that Satan cannot break.

Genuine praise comes from the heart even during times of sorrow, disappointment, discouragement and temptation. The praise of His people brings glory to God. In addition, your praise and worship bring joy to God. He is pleased to hear the voices of His people raised in songs of thanksgiving and praise.

As you complete this study in the First Place program, make a list of the things for which you are most thankful. How has this program helped you in learning about God and praising Him for what He has done for you? Consider how you can continue with your commitment to Bible study, prayer and Scripture memory for your spiritual health, as well as the Live-It plan and exercise for your physical health. May God bless you in your endeavor.

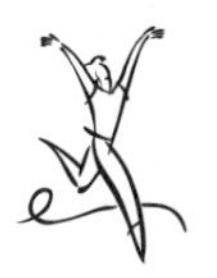

Lord God, let me enter Your gates with thanksgiving and praise. I am thankful and bless Your name for You, O Lord, are good; Your mercy is everlasting and Your truth endures forever (see Psalm 100:4-5).

Father God, I will extol You, my God and King; I will bless Your name for ever and ever. Every day I will bless You and praise You, for great are You, Lord—Your greatness is unfathomable (see Psalm 145:1-3).

Dear Lord, let me continually offer a sacrifice of praise to You. Let it be the fruit of my lips, giving thanks to Your holy name (see Hebrews 13:15).

Note

1. Beth Moore, *Praying God's Word* (Nashville, TN: Broadman and Holman, 2000), pp. 5-7.

Group Prayer Requests Today's Date:________________

Name	Request	Results

DINING OUT— SOUTH OF THE BORDER

Wellness Worksheet One

Mexican food is known for its hot and spicy flavors. Dining south of the border is also popular for its festive atmosphere. Mexican restaurants offer good times and good food. You might think that Mexican food is off limits. Actually, the staples of Mexican cuisine are nutritious choices: chicken and other lean meats, tortillas, beans, rice and salsa. Of course, many also offer less healthy choices such as fried tortillas, refried beans, too much cheese, high-fat dips and sauces and portions that are too large. Be careful or your food fiesta can easily exceed a whole day's worth of calories and fat!

Menu Lingo

To make healthy choices, you must first learn to read the menu.

Low in Fat	High in Fat
Baked, broiled, simmered, or *asada* (grilled)	Fried or crispy
Salsa verde (green sauce)	*Chili con queso* (cheese sauce)
Veracruz or *ranchero* (tomato-based) sauces	Refried, often with lard
Picante sauce or salsa	*Chorizo* (sausage)
Fajitas (grilled meat and soft tortillas)	Guacamole and sour cream

Healthy Choices

Appetizers

How do hot chips with fresh salsa or chili con queso sound? It's easy to consume 500 calories or more before your meal arrives. Plan ahead to limit the number of chips you will eat (five to eight chips are around 100 calories). Better yet, ask that chips not be brought to your table. Ask for steamed corn tortillas instead.

Tortilla or bean soup and a salad are a healthy start to your meal—they can even be the whole meal! Ask for the salad dressing, guacamole and sour cream to be served on the side. Salsa makes a nutritious no-fat dressing. Watch out for taco salad though—particularly if it's served in a tortilla shell.

The Main Meal

Mexican dinners tend to be large. Avoid combination or deluxe plates and order a la carte or side orders instead. Another option is to split a combination plate with a companion.

Choose the following dishes for a healthier meal:

- Grilled chicken breast with rice and vegetables
- Fajitas with grilled chicken or lean meat, but watch out for cheese, guacamole and sour cream; ask for extra lettuce, tomatoes and salsa instead.
- Chicken enchiladas with red or green (*verde*) sauce; hold the sour cream.
- Bean or chicken burritos made with a soft (not fried) tortilla. Request the amount of cheese to be cut in half.

Choose the following dishes less often:

- Tacos, chalupas and flautas
- Cheese enchiladas or enchiladas with cheese or cream sauce
- *Carnitas* (fried beef or pork) or chorizo
- Fried burrito or *chimichanga*

Other Tips

Let family or friends who are dining with you know that you plan to eat healthy. Don't let what others order change your plans for choosing nutritious low-fat and low-calorie foods.

Watch portion sizes; ask for a to-go box before your meal or split your meal with a companion.

Remember, by ordering a la carte items you can pick and choose the foods that are healthiest and that you enjoy. Order a side of Mexican rice and pinto or black beans—instead of refried beans—with your main item.

Become familiar with a few restaurants you enjoy and where you know you can order healthy foods. Make a plan and stick with it. Remember your goal of reaching or maintaining a healthy weight. Avoid restaurants, situations or foods that may knock you off your plan.

Putting It All Together

In the table below list the Mexican restaurants where you dine most often. Next, list the foods that you usually order. Now, what can you do to make your meals healthier? Use this table to help you plan for healthy choices the next time you eat Mexican food.

Restaurant	Usual Choices (Be specific)	Better Choices

No matter whether it's traditional Mexican cuisine, Tex-Mex or Mexican-American, you can enjoy a healthful meal when eating south of the border. The key is having a plan, knowing how to find healthful choices, ordering wisely and eating what you know is best for you.

PRESSING ON TOWARD THE GOAL

Wellness Worksheet Two

But one thing I do: Forgetting what is behind and straining toward what is ahead, I press on toward the goal to win the prize for which God has called me heavenward in Christ Jesus.

Philippians 3:13-14

Two dictionary definitions of "goal": the ending point of a race or the end toward which effort is directed. Too often we focus on the end of the race and forget about the effort. It's easy to set goals; it's much harder to formulate a plan and accomplish the necessary steps to win the prize.

Winning Goals

The Bible makes it clear that goals are an important part of the Christian life. Philippians 3:13-14 is one example. Why are goals so important? Because in life we need goals to help us achieve. God clearly desires to be at the center of all our plans (see Proverbs 3:5-6; 16:9). When setting goals, the most important question we must ask ourselves is, *Is my goal in line with God's desire for my life?*

When setting lifestyle goals, consider the goal worthwhile and consistent with God's plan for your life (see Mark 12:28-31) if you can answer yes to one or more of the following questions:

- Will achieving my goal help me grow closer to God and serve Him better?
- Will achieving my goal help me to feel better about myself and live more effectively?
- Will achieving my goal improve my ability to serve others?
- Will achieving my goal improve my health and well-being?

Prayerfully seek God's wisdom and guidance before moving ahead with your goals and plans. You should also seek wise counsel from trusted family and friends. Remember, it's better to spend several weeks prayerfully considering and developing your goals and plans than it is to start tomorrow toward a goal that you can't (or shouldn't) achieve.

Setting Realistic Goals

How many times have you made up your mind that you were going to make a change and then fallen short of your goal? Do any of these sound familiar?

- I'll never eat dessert again.
- I'm going to exercise at 7 A.M. every day.
- I'm going to spend one hour daily in quiet time.
- I will lose 60 pounds in three months.

It's best to avoid setting too rigid or all-or-none goals that use words such as "never again," "always," "every day," "must," etc. Setting goals that are unrealistic or too demanding will set you up for failure and disappointment.

Another reason people often fall short of their goals is that they try to take on too much too soon. Realistic goals and a well-thought-out plan are the most important ingredients for success.

Setting Goals and Developing a Plan

The key to setting goals and building a successful plan is to ask yourself the right questions.

What Do You Want to Accomplish?

It's important to have a clear idea of where you want to go before you get started. Do you really want to achieve a certain weight or is the underlying issue that you want to feel better about yourself? When setting a goal, it's important to have a clear idea of the benefits you are looking for. Ask yourself how your life will be different when you achieve your goal. How will you feel if you don't achieve your goal?

What Are Your Motivations?

People who are successful in achieving and maintaing long-term goals have clear reasons for doing so. In other words, the reward has to be worth the effort. When setting goals, it's much more important to focus on things you can do rather than on things you wish you could be. Motivations such as improving your relationships, feeling better and improving your health are much stronger motivations than looking better or achieving an ideal body weight for a special event such as a high school reunion or wedding.

What Steps Do You Need to Take?

When setting goals it's important to have the long-term results in mind, but it's much more important to focus on what you can do each day to achieve them. It's much better to start with small goals and succeed than to start with big goals and fail because it is too overwhelming. With each success, you'll gain the confidence and encouragement you need to take the next step.

What Things Might Keep You from Reaching Your Goal?

It's important to think about situations, people and feelings that may keep you from achieving or maintaining your goals. Understanding your past successes or failures is a great place to start when setting new goals. Think about some goals you've set for yourself in the past. What worked for you and what didn't? Are you committed to achieving your goal? Are you willing to stick with your plans when times get tough or you experience a setback? It's also important to have goals and plans that are flexible. You will en-counter life changes along the way; be prepared to adjust your expectations.

Who Can Help and How Can They Help You?

It's very difficult to make lifestyle changes without the support of family and friends. Having a solid system of support greatly increases your chances for success. Try to seek out people who have accomplished what you are trying to achieve. Finding family and friends who have goals similar to yours can also be helpful. This step requires some effort on your part; you will have to ask for the help you need. Don't expect people to understand your needs and volunteer their help.

How Can You Monitor Your Progress?

Self-monitoring is one of the best predictors of success when striving for a goal. The ability to see your progress along the way helps keep you motivated and on track. The path to most goals is usually not a straight line. By monitoring your progress you'll see that a slip up or two along the way can't reverse all the progress you've made. When setting goals, make sure you build in a plan for monitoring your progress. Have a plan for rewarding yourself as you achieve important victories along the way.

> "If you don't know what you're aiming for, you'll hit it every time."

> "If you keep on doing the things you've always done, you'll keep getting the things you've always gotten."

Wellness Worksheet Three

PREVENTING DIABETES

Diabetes is a serious disease and is the seventh leading cause of death in the United States. Sixteen million Americans have diabetes, and one in three don't even know they have it! Each year, nearly 800,000 people are diagnosed and over 190,000 deaths result from diabetes. Diabetes kills more women each year than breast cancer. Diabetes is very damaging to the body and is a major cause of blindness, kidney disease, nerve damage and amputations. People with diabetes have two to four times the risk of heart attack and stroke.

Types of Diabetes

Diabetes means that your blood sugar—glucose—is too high. Your blood always has some sugar in it because your body requires a constant supply of sugar for energy. However, too much sugar in the blood is not good for your health. Most of the food you eat is converted into glucose—sugar—for energy. For the glucose to get into the body's cells, a hormone called insulin must be present. In a person who has diabetes, either the body does not produce enough insulin or the cells don't use it properly. As a result, blood sugar levels rise. There are two major types of diabetes.

- **Type 1 Diabetes** is an autoimmune disease in which the body does not produce enough insulin. It usually begins in childhood or young adulthood. Without enough insulin, the body cannot control blood sugar. The only way to survive with type 1 diabetes is to take daily injections of insulin. Type 1 accounts for only 5 to 10 percent of all diabetes sufferers.
- **Type 2 Diabetes** results from an inability to make enough insulin or properly use it—insulin resistance. Type 2 is the most common form of diabetes and accounts for 90 to 95 percent of cases. This form of diabetes usually develops in adults over the age of 45. Nearly 80 percent of people with type 2 diabetes are overweight. Type 2 diabetes is on the rise due to the increasing age, weight and sedentary lifestyles of Americans.

Risk Factors for Type 2 Diabetes

Doctors don't yet understand all the reasons people develop type 2 diabetes. The following factors—many of which can be lowered with healthy lifestyle habits—are associated with a higher risk:

- Family history of type 2 diabetes in a parent or sibling
- Overweight and obesity (ideal body weight ≥ 120% or a body mass index ≥ 27)
- A history of diabetes during pregnancy or delivery of a baby weighing more than nine pounds
- Low HDL cholesterol (≤ 35 mg/dL) or high trigycerides (≥ 250 mg/dL)
- High blood pressure (≥ 140/90)
- African American, Hispanic and Native American descent
- A sedentary lifestyle

Diagnoses

Experts now recommend that adults 45 years and older be tested for diabetes. If you're under 45 years of age and you have one or more risk factors for diabetes, you should also be tested. Early diagnosis and treatment can lower the risk of the serious complications associated with diabetes. The best way to test for diabetes is to have a blood test performed after you haven't eaten anything for at least eight hours. This is called a fasting plasma glucose test. Do you know your blood sugar level?

Risk Classification	Fasting Plasma Glucose Level	My Level
Normal	<110 mg/dL	
Increased Risk	110 to 125 mg/dL	
Diabetes	≥126 mg/dL	

If your blood glucose is normal, take lifestyle steps to keep it that way and have repeat testing every three years. If your level puts you at an increased risk, ask your doctor about further testing. If you have diabetes, you need to take your blood sugar levels very seriously. If you have diabetes, you need to work with your doctor and a registered dietician to do all you can to keep your blood sugar under control.

Prevention

There are several things you can do to lower your risk for type 2 diabetes. If you're at risk, it's important that you do all you can to prevent diabetes. Fortunately, following the First Place lifestyle will help you keep your risk low. In addition to a healthy lifestyle, make sure to get regular medical checkups.

- **Follow a Healthy Eating Plan**
  Healthy eating can help to keep your risk low. The most important thing is to maintain a healthy body weight. A healthy eating plan is high in fruits, vegetables and whole grains, and low in foods that are high in fat, saturated fat and cholesterol.
- **Control Your Weight**
  Weight gain is associated with increasing risk for diabetes—the higher your weight, the higher your risk. If you're overweight, a weight loss of as little as 10 percent can significantly reduce your chances of developing diabetes. Achieving and maintaining your healthy weight range will help you keep your risk even lower.
- **Exercise Regularly**
  A sedentary lifestyle and low level of physical fitness is associated with an increased risk for developing diabetes. Regular physical activity and exercise helps your body use insulin and sugar more efficiently. Physical activity also helps you achieve and maintain your healthy weight and lowers your risk for heart disease. Are you fitting in at least 30 minutes of physical activity several days each week?

SPORTS AND RECREATIONAL ACTIVITIES

Wellness Worksheet Four

There are many different ways to fit physical activity into your lifestyle. The first step is to find activities you enjoy. Then you need to get out there and do them on a regular basis. Sports and recreational activities can be a great way to fit in physical activity. Check out the following benefits:

- They strengthen muscles, burn calories and reduce stress just as well as other types of exercise.
- They provide opportunities to enjoy your health and fitness. Playing and having fun helps you stay young and keeps you motivated.
- They allow you to spend time with family and friends and meet new people too! Remember, relationships are just as important to your overall health and well-being as exercise and good nutrition.
- The competitive nature of some sports can inspire you to set fitness goals and stay motivated. Setting a goal such as finishing a 10K race or playing in a tennis league can make your workouts more meaningful.

Select Recreational Activities You Enjoy

No matter what your skill, coordination or fitness level, you can find activities that you can enjoy. Find one or two sports or recreational activities you enjoy, and fit them into your fitness routine one to three times each week. Consider the following list of possibilities:

Badminton
Basketball
Bike rallies
Fun runs/walks
Golf
Hiking
Racquetball
Skating
Skiing
Soccer
Softball
Squash
Tennis
Volleyball

Individual Sports and Activities

- **Fun Runs/Walks**: Many people enjoy participating in local fun runs or walks. These community events offer challenge and camaraderie. Most people don't run to compete with others; their goal is to finish the race and feel good about their accomplishment. Training for a local event is a great way to keep you motivated and break up your exercise routine. Joining a walking or running group is a great way to meet other people with similar interests.

- **Bike Rallies**: If you enjoy bicycling, you might want to train for a bike rally. Bike rallies are generally anywhere from 25 to 100 miles long. Choose your distance and start training. Training for a rally is a great motivator. Participating in a rally provides a great source of accomplishment and is a fun way to meet other people. Well-organized rides attract thousands of riders of all fitness levels and create a fun and exciting environment. Most cities also have bicycle clubs that get together on the weekends for longer rides and fellowship. *Never do a longer event, whether walking, running or cycling, without proper training.*

- **Skating**: There are several ways to skate these days. The two most popular ways are in-line skating—roller-blading—and ice-skating. Actually, inline skating is one of the fastest growing recreational activities in this country. Skating is a great aerobic exercise and a good way to burn calories. Skating does take a little more skill than walking, jogging or bicycling, and the risk of injury is much higher. Before making the investment, rent a pair of skates and take formal lessons. When inline skating, wear wrist guards, protective padding and a helmet.

- **Skiing**: Many people have the opportunity to go downhill skiing one or more times each year. The annual ski trip can be a great motivator to keep yourself in shape. To ski enjoyably and safely you need a moderate to high level of cardiovascular endurance, muscular fitness, flexibility, balance and coordination. Spend at least two or three months getting yourself in condition to go skiing. The risk of injury during skiing is very high, and the injuries can be severe: broken bones and torn ligaments. High altitude and cold temperatures are also important safety considerations.

- **Golf:** Golf is a popular sport that provides a great opportunity to enjoy the outdoors. Golf is more of a game of skill than it is of physical fitness. However, by walking and carrying your own clubs, golf can count toward your weekly physical activity goal. Physical fitness can improve your game. To be successful in golf, focus on three components of fitness: strength/power, flexibility and cardiovascular endurance. Cardiovascular endurance is essential to help keep your energy up during a long round of golf. Flexibility exercises increase your range of motion and prevent injury. Muscular fitness can improve the power and speed of your swing.

Racquet Sports

Racquet sports such as tennis, racquetball and squash are popular and can be played as singles or doubles. All of them offer a moderate to vigorous workout, depending on the intensity you put into it. Playing singles usually requires more effort and burns more calories. In addition to providing health and fitness benefits, you will also develop balance, agility and coordination. The more fit you are the better you'll play. Develop a regular fitness routine to help improve your game and lower your risk of injury. You need cardiovascular endurance, flexibility and strength to play your best.

For equipment all you need to play is a good pair of shoes, a racquet (or just your hand for handball), a partner and a court. Shoes are probably your most important piece of equipment. You'll need a good court shoe with adequate cushioning. You'll also need good heel and ankle support because these sports have a lot of side-to-side movement. Many of the sports require protective eyewear. Check with a YMCA, local fitness club or recreation center to sign up for lessons, or a local racquet club to improve your game and meet other people.

Team Sports

Team sports such as basketball, softball, volleyball and soccer have both fitness and social benefits. They can be light, moderate or vigorous in intensity depending on the sport and how hard you play. Regardless of the intensity, including team sports in your fitness program can offer a variety of benefits. Low intensity sports such as softball and volleyball are a great outlet for competition and fellowship. Regardless of the sport you choose, the more fit you are the better you'll play. You need cardiovascular endurance, muscular fitness and flexibility to play your best.

Be careful if you play team sports only sporadically. It's easy to let the competitive drive take over and overexert yourself—the weekend-warrior syndrome. Some sports can take a greater toll on your body, especially as you grow older. Make sure you wear the appropriate shoes and protective gear. As you would for any exercise, spend some time warming up with light activity and stretching before playing. Cool down gradually after playing vigorous sports such as basketball or soccer.

STAYING ACTIVE WHILE TRAVELING

Wellness Worksheet Five

Almost everyone travels—whether it's for business, a weekend getaway or a family vacation. Many people find it more difficult to stay physically active while on the road. The good news is that with a little planning, you can enjoy the benefits of physical activity while traveling. Sure, it may be a little harder to make time for physical activity when you travel, but the benefits will be well worth the effort.

Physical Activity on a Business Trip

When traveling for business, sometimes it's hard to make your own schedule—schedules are tight, meetings run late, flights are delayed and colleagues often want to entertain you. The key to a physically active business trip is—you guessed it—planning! Try the following tips for fitting in activity when you travel on business:

- Rise a little earlier in the morning to fit in some activity; this way you can't miss it!
- Schedule activity into your day just like you do for meetings.
- Make sure colleagues know that physical activity is important to you.
- When traveling, wear comfortable shoes or carry tennis shoes in your carry-on bag. Walk between meetings or while waiting for your flight—even 10 minutes will help.
- Fit in activity by taking the stairs instead of the elevator, carrying your own bags and walking wherever you can.

Physical Activity on Vacation

Traveling for pleasure is a great way to enjoy your health and fitness: hike in the mountains, walk along a secluded beach, bicycle through the countryside or windsurf over the waves. Don't think so much about following your usual routine; look for new ways to be physically active. When you're planning your trip, take time to plan ways to fit activity into your schedule. Check out the following ideas for active travel:

- Local attractions such as parks, zoos, nature trails and other activities can provide opportunities to see the sights and get some activity at the same time!
- Planning ahead allows you to take clothing, shoes and equipment you will need for physical activity.
- Plan active vacations, such as hiking or camping. Stay at hotels with exercise facilities.
- Try to find ways to be active with your traveling companions: rent bicycles, skates or other recreational equipment. It's often easier to stay active if you have the support of others.
- Find out about the weather conditions before you go so you can pack the right clothing.
- Take along recreational equipment such as tennis or racquetball racquets, golf clubs, a jump rope or other things you enjoy.

Healthful Tips for Active Travelers

Check with the Hotel Where You Will Be Staying

- Does it provide an exercise room?
- Are there safe walking paths nearby?
- Is there a mall nearby where you can walk?
- Are there local fitness facilities you can use?
- Pack a swimsuit and take advantage of the hotel pool.

Be Prepared for Changes in Plans

- If the weather is bad, walk in a mall or go to an indoor fitness center.
- For a quick workout, take along elastic exercise bands, hand weights, a jump rope, music or an exercise video for activity in your hotel room.
- If a flight is delayed, take a brisk walk around the airport terminal.

You may need to lower your expectations when traveling—even 10 minutes of activity is beneficial. Don't skip activity just because you can't do your usual routine.

Avoid overdoing it. You want to be rested and relaxed when you travel. Don't push yourself when you're tired. Sometimes rest will do you more good than exercise. Don't let trying to fit in a workout become another stress when you travel. There's plenty of time for physical activity when you get home.

Doing your activity first thing in the morning is a great way to fit it in. This way if a meeting runs late, a flight is delayed or something else comes up, you've done your activity for the day.

While traveling, try to get plenty of sleep, drink lots of water and eat healthful foods. Carry healthy snacks with you when you travel. A little snack can give you the boost you need to make it to the next meal. If you get too hungry, you may opt for eating out rather than working out!

- What are some things you can do to fit activity into your next trip?

Wellness Worksheet Six

TAKE TIME FOR A HEALTHY LUNCH

Do you take time for lunch? Our busy lifestyles often lead to lunch on the run. For many, lunch is a popular social time rather than a time to nourish the body. Some of us are so busy we don't even take time for lunch.

The most popular lunchtime fares are sandwiches, hamburgers and salads. The truth of the matter is that traditional sandwiches and salads may not be any lower in fat and calories than the fast-food burger!

Avoiding lunch leads to fatigue, hunger and overeating later in the day or night. Extreme hunger can also lead to cravings for junk food and binge eating. On the positive side, a nutritious lunch can give your body the fuel it needs to meet the physical and mental demands of the rest of the day. Lunchtime can also offer a much needed break after a hard morning of work. A light nutritious meal plus 10 to 20 minutes of moderate activity during the lunch hour is a great way to achieve good health and a healthy weight. Eating too much fat, calories and sugar may do you in for the rest of the day.

Excuses for Not Eating a Healthy Lunch

- No time! Even if you can't stop for a relaxing lunch break, you can take a few minutes to eat some nutritious foods. It's easy to eat a sandwich, cheese and crackers, yogurt or fresh fruit—if you have prepared ahead of time.

- I don't need the calories! This is *not* a good reason to skip lunch. Your body needs energy and nutrients throughout the day. Skipping meals only leads to overeating later in the day. With every meal you skip, you rob your body of important nutrients and sources for the energy needed to make it through the afternoon hours.

Examine your reasons for not eating a healthy lunch. What are some possible solutions? What are the benefits of eating a nutritious lunch? Begin making plans to make a nutritious lunch a regular part of your day.

Eating Out

Eating a healthy lunch is now easier than ever. Fast food and other restaurants now offer several nutritious and low-fat options. Of course, most menus offer selections that are high in calories, fat and cholesterol, and low in fresh fruits, vegetables and whole-grains. The key is to plan ahead and order what you know is best.

Best Bets for a Healthy Lunch

- A fresh salad with an assortment of colorful vegetables, low-fat dressing *(On the side please!)*, grilled chicken, grilled chicken sandwich *(Hold the mayo!)*, bean and cheese burrito *(Go easy on the cheese and add extra lettuce and tomato!)*, small hamburger or baked potato *(Toppings on the side!)* are all good choices. All these meals have fewer than 400 calories and 30 percent or less fat.

- Deli sandwiches can be a healthy choice. Choose lean meats such as turkey, ham or roast beef. Ask for mustard or light mayonnaise. Ask for less meat (usually half the typical serving), more lettuce, tomato and other vegetables, and whole grain bread. Hold the chips or fries.

- Pizza can be a good choice if you choose carefully. Stick to vegetable pizza and ask for less cheese and more sauce and vegetables. Limit yourself to one or two slices of thin crust pizza. Eat a salad too.

- Pick out three or four restaurants where you can get healthy foods. Suggest to friends and colleagues that you eat at these places when you eat out for lunch.

Worst Bets for a Healthy Lunch

- A hamburger and fries, a tuna salad sandwich or a chicken Caesar salad can supply half of the fat and calories recommended for an entire day. The typical deli-style sandwich piled with meat, mayonnaise and cheese—and bacon if it's a club sandwich—is not any better.

- Is salad a healthy choice? A ladle of regular salad dressing contains four tablespoons—nearly 300 calories of fat or half of your recommended daily intake.

- Fried foods—french fries, fried chicken and fish, burgers, tacos, etc.—should not be a regular part of the lunchtime meal. Frying can double the fat and calories.

- Portion sizes can be two to three times what you need—split a meal with a companion or take some home to eat for another meal.

Packing Your Lunch

Packing a healthy lunch starts with planning. A healthy brown-bag lunch starts in the grocery store. Plan ahead to buy a variety of nutritious foods that you enjoy and are convenient for you to prepare and pack along. When preparing your lunch, remember the key principles of variety, balance and moderation.

- You'll need an assortment of plastic containers, plastic bags and maybe even a thermos. An insulated lunch bag or cooler can keep foods cool if you don't have access to a refrigerator.
- Canned and frozen fruits, vegetables and beans can be placed in individual-sized plastic containers. You can do the same with soups. Add your own seasonings when packing. Your meal is now ready to heat in a microwave when you're ready.
- Take along low-fat dairy foods. Milk can be kept cool in a thermos and yogurt can stay at room temperature for several hours. Mix canned fruit or fresh vegetables with cottage cheese in a plastic container.
- Keep plenty of your favorite fruits and vegetables on hand wherever you are. If they need cutting or peeling, do it the night before. Better yet, prepare them as soon as you come home from the grocery store. Store them away in plastic bags or containers so they're ready to go when you are.
- Make a sandwich with lean meat and fresh vegetables the night before. Place it in a sandwich container or plastic bag and it will be ready to go when you leave in the morning.
- Make lunch quick and easy by bringing leftovers. Most leftovers can be easily reheated in a microwave. When cooking at home, make extra portions and store the extras individually for a ready-to-serve lunch.

- Packing your own lunch also saves money; it's much cheaper to pack your own than to eat out. The savings over an entire year could pay for a health club membership or home exercise equipment!
- Always have enjoyable standbys when you find yourself short on time or choices. Dried and canned soups and fruits, crackers, peanut butter, oatmeal, cereal, bagels and energy bars can be kept on hand in a pantry or desk drawer for a quick and easy lunch anytime.

List some things you're ready to try for a more healthy lunch whether you eat out or pack your own.

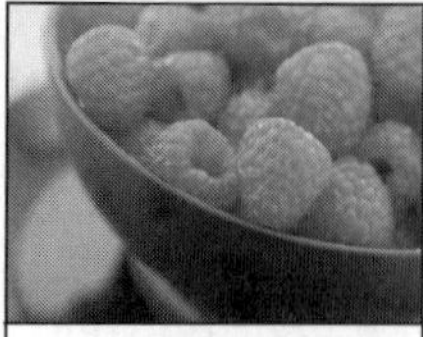

Pressing On to the Prize

FIRST PLACE MENU PLANS

Each plan is based on approximately 1400 calories.

Breakfast	2 breads, 1 fruit, 1 milk, 0-½ fat (When a meat exchange is used, milk is omitted.)
Lunch	2 meats, 2 breads, 1 vegetable, 1 fruit, 1 fat
Dinner	3 meats, 2 breads, 2 vegetables, 1 fat
Snacks	1 bread, 1 fruit, 1 milk, ½-1 fat (or any remaining exchanges)

For more calories, add the following to the 1400 calorie plan.

1600 calories	2 breads, 1 fat
1800 calories	2 meats, 3 breads, 1 vegetable, 1 fat
2000 calories	2 meats, 4 breads, 1 vegetable, 3 fats
2200 calories	2 meats, 5 breads, 1 vegetable, 1 fruit, 5 fats
2400 calories	2 meats, 6 breads, 2 vegetables, 1 fruit, 6 fats

The exchanges for these meals were calculated using the MasterCook software. It uses a database of over 6,000 food items prepared using United States Department of Agriculture (USDA) publications and information from food manufacturers. As with any nutritional program, MasterCook calculates the nutritional values of the recipes based on ingredients. Nutrition may vary due to how the food is prepared, where the food comes from, i.e., geography, soil content, season, ripeness, processing and method of preparation. For these reasons, please use the recipes and menu plans as approximate guides. As always, consult your physician and/or a registered dietician before starting a diet program.

Menu Plans for Two Weeks

Breakfasts

2 low-fat Eggo waffles
½ c. applesauce, sweetened with
1 package Sweet & Low and
2 tbsp. raisins
1 c. nonfat milk

Exchanges: 2 breads, 2 fruits, 1 milk, ½ fat

~~~~~~

1 package flavored instant oatmeal (no sugar added)
2 walnut halves, chopped
1 small banana
1 c. nonfat milk

Exchanges: 2 breads, 1 fruit, 1 milk, ½ fat

~~~~~~

1 small reduced-fat oat muffin
1 medium fresh peach or other fruit
1 c. artificially sweetened, nonfat fruit-flavored yogurt

Exchanges: 2 breads, 1 fruit, 1 milk, ½ fat

~~~~~~

¾ c. Rice Chex
½ English muffin
½ tsp. reduced-fat margarine
1 tsp. all-fruit spread
1 c. nonfat milk
1 small banana

Exchanges: 2 breads, 1 fruit, 1 milk, ¼ fat

~~~~~~

⅓ medium cantaloupe or honeydew
1 c. artificially sweetened, nonfat pineapple-flavored yogurt
¼ c. Grape Nuts

Exchanges: 2 breads, 1 fruit, 1 milk

~~~~~~
~~~~~~

Brunch Casserole

- 4 slices wheat bread, crusts removed
- 2 oz. turkey sausage
- ¼ c. mushrooms, chopped
- 1 tsp. onion, chopped
- 4 eggs, beaten (or 1 c. egg substitute)
- 1 c. nonfat milk
- ¼ tsp. salt
- ⅛ tsp. black pepper
- ⅛ tsp. granulated garlic
- 2 oz. 2% cheddar cheese, shredded
- Nonstick cooking spray

Line bottom of 9x9-inch casserole dish with bread. Spray skillet with nonstick cooking spray. Sauté sausage until done. Remove from skillet and set aside. Sauté mushrooms and onions until tender. Crumble sausage and combine with mushrooms and onion. Sprinkle mixture over bread. Combine eggs, milk and seasonings and pour over top. Sprinkle with cheese. Cover and refrigerate overnight. Before cooking, set out for 15 minutes. Bake at 350° F 40 to 45 minutes. Serves 4.

Serve each with ½ grapefruit.

Exchanges: 2 meats, 1 bread, 1 fruit, ¼ milk, ½ fat

~~~~~~

- 1 slice whole-wheat (or 2 slices diet multigrain) bread, toasted
- 2 tsp. all-fruit spread
- 1 c. nonfat plain yogurt, artificially sweetened, garnished with
- 3 tbsp. wheat germ (or 2 tbsp. Grape Nuts)
- 6 oz. orange juice

Exchanges: 2 breads, 1 fruit, 1 milk

~~~~~~

- 1 c. Kellogg's Nutri-Grain cereal
- 1 c. nonfat milk
- 2 tbsp. raisins

Exchanges: 1½ breads, 1 fruit, 1 milk

~~~~~~

Breakfast Pita

- 1 6-inch whole-wheat pocket pita
- ¼ c. 2% cottage cheese
- ⅓ c. diced peaches, in own juice
- 2 walnuts, chopped
~~~~~~

Combine cottage cheese, peaches and walnuts. Split pita in half; fill each half with cottage cheese mixture.

Exchanges: **1 meat, 2 breads, 1 fruit, 1 fat**

~~~~~~

Breakfast Burrito

2 6-inch fat-free flour tortillas
½ c. egg substitute, scrambled
2 tbsp. onion, chopped
2 tbsp. bell pepper, chopped
2 tbsp. salsa
Serve with 1 small orange.

Exchanges: **1 meat, 2 breads, ½ vegetable, 1 fruit, ½ fat**

~~~~~~

1 2-oz. whole-wheat bagel
1 tbsp. reduced-calorie cream cheese
3 medium stewed prunes (or 3 plums)
1 c. nonfat milk

Exchanges: **2 breads, 1 fruit, 1 milk, ½ fat**

~~~~~~

1 c. oatmeal with
¼ tsp. reduced-fat margarine
Dash cinnamon
Dash nutmeg
2 tbsp. raisins
1 c. nonfat milk

Exchanges: **1½ breads, 1 fruit, 1 milk, ½ fat**

~~~~~~

3 4-inch low-fat pancakes
1 tsp. strawberry all-fruit spread
½ c. fresh strawberries, chopped
6 oz. nonfat plain yogurt

Pancake topping: Melt strawberry spread and combine with fresh strawberries and yogurt.

Exchanges: **2 breads, 1 fruit, 1 milk**

~~~~~~
~~~~~~

Broiled Chicken Breasts

2.5-oz. boneless, skinless chicken breast, broiled
and served with mixed bean salad:
1 c. cut Italian green beans, cooked
1 c. wax beans
1 c. chickpeas, drained
1 tbsp. reduced-fat Italian dressing

Serve each with 2 breadsticks, ½ teaspoon margarine and 1 small nectarine.

Exchanges: 2 meats, 2 breads, 1½ vegetables, 1 fruit, 1 fat

~~~~~~

Mozzarella Sandwich

2 oz. reduced-fat mozzarella cheese
¼ c. romaine lettuce leaves
¼ c. roasted red bell pepper, cut into strips
2 slices tomato
1 tsp. red wine vinegar
1½ tsp. lite Italian dressing
2 1-oz. slices Italian bread, toasted
1 c. whole green beans, cooked and chilled

Drizzle vinegar and dressing over bell peppers and tomato slices. Layer cheese, lettuce, bell pepper and tomato between bread slices.

Serve with 1 small orange.

Exchanges: 2 meats, 2 breads, 2 vegetables, 1 fruit, 1 fat

~~~~~~

Egg Salad Sandwich

1 egg, hard-boiled and minced
1 egg white, hard-boiled and minced
¼ c. celery, chopped
¼ c. red onion, chopped
2 tsp. reduced-calorie mayonnaise
2 slices reduced-calorie rye bread

Combine minced eggs, celery, onion and mayonnaise. Spread on bread to make sandwich.

Serve with 1 cup each carrot sticks and zucchini, 2 tablespoons reduced-fat ranch dressing and 4 ounces sugar-free, nonfat, chocolate-flavored frozen yogurt.

Exchanges: 1½ meats, 2 breads, 2 vegetables, 1 fat

~~~~~~

Soup and Salad

1 8-oz. can vegetable soup (90-calorie), served with
2 c. mixed green lettuce
½ c. roasted red bell pepper strips, chilled
½ c. celery, sliced
2 oz. reduced-fat cheddar cheese, diced
1 tbsp. lite Italian dressing
1 1-oz. slice Italian or French bread
1 tsp. reduced-fat margarine

Serve with 20 oyster crackers and 1 cup strawberries.

Exchanges: 2 meats, 2½ breads, 2 vegetables, 1 fat

~~~~~~

Spinach, Bean and Chicken Salad

2 c. torn spinach leaves
¼ c. cooked cannellini (white kidney) beans, drained
2 oz. skinless, boneless chicken breast, cooked and diced
2 tbsp. reduced-fat Catalina-style dressing

Serve with ½ cup each carrot and celery sticks, 2 long breadsticks and 2 small plums.

Exchanges: 2 meats, 2 breads, 2 vegetables, 1 fruit, ½ fat

~~~~~~

Burger King Kid's Meal

1 small hamburger (without mayonnaise)
1 small French fries
1 small diet soda

Serve with 1 small apple.

Exchanges: 1½ meats, 2½ breads, 1 fruit, 2 fats

~~~~~~

1 10- to 11-oz. frozen light dinner entrée (with 300 to 350 calories, fewer than 800 mg. sodium and fewer than 10 grams fat)
Spinach salad with mushrooms
1 tbsp. reduced-calorie dressing
Serve with 15 grapes.

Exchanges: 1 ½ meats, 2 breads, 1 vegetable, 1 fruit, ½ fat

Chicken Salad Sandwich

2 oz. cooked skinless, boneless chicken breast, chopped
¼ c. celery, chopped
2 tsp. reduced-calorie mayonnaise
Pinch freshly ground black pepper
2 romaine lettuce leaves
2 slices tomato
2 slices reduced-calorie whole-wheat bread

Combine chicken, celery, mayonnaise and black pepper for sandwich filling. Spread on bread slices. Top with tomato and lettuce.

Serve with ½ cup each cucumber slices and carrot sticks, 1 small banana and ½ cup reduced-calorie vanilla pudding (made with nonfat milk).

Exchanges: 2 meats, 1 ½ breads, 1 vegetable, 1 fruit, ½ milk

Roast Beef Sandwich

1 ½ oz. cooked lean, boneless roast beef, thinly sliced
2 slices reduced-calorie bread
2 slices tomato
2 romaine lettuce leaves
1 tbsp. reduced-fat Thousand Island dressing

Serve with ½ cup each celery and carrot sticks, and 1 cup sugar-free white-grape flavored gelatin mixed with 1 cup grapes.

Exchanges: 1 ½ meats, 1 bread, 1 vegetable, 1 fruit, ½ fat

Cheese and Veggie Sandwich with Tomato Soup

1 8-oz. can ready-to-eat tomato soup
2 slices reduced-calorie whole-wheat bread

¼ c. alfalfa sprouts
¼ c. spinach leaves
¼ c. roasted red bell pepper strips, drained
1 oz. slice reduced-fat Swiss cheese
1 tbsp. reduced-fat Thousand Island dressing

Serve with 6 saltine crackers, 1 cup broccoli florets and 1 cup aspartame-sweetened raspberry-flavored nonfat yogurt topped with ½ cup raspberries.

Exchanges: 1 meat, 2 breads, 1 vegetable, 1 fruit, 1 milk, ½ fat

~~~~~~

1 8-oz. can beef barley soup
6 saltine crackers
Dark green salad with vegetables and
1 tbsp. reduced-fat dressing

Serve with 2 slices pineapple, packed in own juice.

Exchanges: 2 meats, 2 breads, 1 vegetable, 1 fruit, ½ fat

~~~~~~

Arby's Turkey Deluxe Sandwich

Green salad with fat-free dressing

Serve with ¼ cup canned peach slices, packed in own juice.

Exchanges: 2½ meats, 2 breads, 1 vegetable, 1 fruit, ½ fat

~~~~~~

Subway Cold Cut Combo

6-inch sandwich loaded with veggies (no mayonnaise or cheese)

Serve with 1 cup mixed berries and substitute 1 bag baked potato chips for ½ of sandwich bread, if desired.

Exchanges: 2 meats, 2½ breads, 1 vegetable, 1 fruit

~~~~~~

2 oz. grilled fat-free frankfurter
1 2-oz. frankfurter bread roll
1 tsp. pickle relish
1 tsp. prepared mustard
1 c. green and red cabbage, shredded
1½ tsp. reduced-fat coleslaw dressing
1 c. carrot sticks

Serve with 1 small apple.

Exchanges: 2 meats, 2 breads, 2 vegetables, 1 fruit, ½ fat

~~~~~~
~~~~~~

Italian Breaded Snapper

- 1 lb. red snapper, cut into 4 fillets
- 1 tbsp. fresh lemon or lime juice
- ½ tsp. salt
- ½ c. Italian-seasoned bread crumbs
- 1 tbsp. olive oil

Rinse fish fillets and pat dry with paper towel. Combine bread crumbs with salt in small plate. Dip fillets in lemon or lime juice; then dip in bread crumbs to coat. Heat oil in large nonstick skillet. Cook fillets over medium heat 4 to 5 minutes each side, turning once (about 10 minutes total for 1-inch thick fillets, or until flaky when tested with fork). Serves 4.

Serve each with 1 cup steamed broccoli, ½ cup cooked pasta tossed with ¼ cup prepared marinara sauce, 1 breadstick and 1 cup mixed berries.

Exchanges: 3 meats, 2 breads, 1½ vegetables, 1 fruit, ½ fat

~~~~~~

Honey-Mustard Pecan Tilapia

- 4 4-oz. tilapia, catfish or similar fish fillets
- ¼ c. Creole or brown mustard
- 2 tbsp. nonfat milk
- 1 tsp. honey
- ¾ c. pecans, or pecan meal, crushed
- Nonstick cooking spray

Preheat oven to 450° F and coat baking sheet with nonstick cooking spray. Rinse fillets and pat dry. Combine mustard, milk and honey in small bowl. Dip fillets in milk mixture; then press into pecans to coat. Bake 12 minutes or until crisp. Serves 4.

Serve each with ¾ cup mashed potatoes, 1 cup green beans and ¾ cup mixed melon balls.

Exchanges: 3 meats, 2 breads, 1 vegetable, 1 fruit, 1 fat

~~~~~~

Ground Beef Stroganoff on Noodles

- 6 oz. egg-free noodles
- 1 c. beef broth
- 1 lb. extra-lean ground beef
- 1 tbsp. reduced-fat margarine
- 1 medium onion, diced
- 8 oz. mushrooms, sliced
- 1 tsp. flour
- ½ tsp. salt
- ½ tsp. ground pepper
- ¾ c. reduced-fat sour cream

Cook noodles according to package directions (omitting salt and fat); then drain and combine with ½ cup beef broth in medium cooking pot. Cook ground beef in skillet over medium heat until well-done. Drain and remove from skillet; set aside. Sauté onions and mushrooms in margarine for 3 minutes, or until tender crisp. Sprinkle with flour and season with salt and pepper. Add remaining beef broth and bring mixture to a boil. Simmer for 2 minutes. Add cooked ground beef and slowly stir in sour cream. Return to heat and cook over low heat until warm—*do not* let boil or sour cream will curdle. Serve over noodles. Serves 4.

Serve each with a spinach salad with ¼ cup sliced strawberries and 1 tablespoon reduced-fat sweet and sour dressing.

Exchanges: 3 meats, 2 breads, 1 vegetable, ¼ fruit, 1 fat

~~~~~~

1 10- to 11-oz. frozen dinner entrée
Tossed salad with veggies and 1 to 2 tbsp. reduced-fat dressing
1 frozen 100% juice bar

Exchanges: 1½ meats, 2 breads, 1 vegetable, 1 fruit, ½ fat

~~~~~~

Pizza Hut Supreme Pizza

2 slices medium Thin and Crispy Supreme
Tossed salad with 1 tbsp. salad dressing
Serve with 1 cup sliced peaches, drained.

Exchanges: 3 meats, 3 breads, 1 vegetable, 1 fruit, 2 fats

~~~~~~

Pork Chops with Cherry Sauce

4 4-oz. boneless, center-cut pork chops, trimmed of fat
½ tsp. garlic salt
½ tsp. ground pepper
1 16-oz. bag frozen dark red pitted cherries, thawed and drained
¾ tsp. dried leaf oregano, crushed
½ tsp. ground nutmeg
½ tsp. balsamic vinegar
½ c. red grape juice
Nonstick cooking spray

Coat a large skillet with nonstick cooking spray. Coat pork chops evenly on both sides with garlic and pepper. Arrange in preheated skillet and brown well on both sides over medium heat. Combine grape juice, vinegar, remaining seasonings and half of cherries in blender. Puree and pour over
~~~~~~

pork chops in skillet. Sprinkle remaining cherries over top; then reduce heat. Cover and simmer 10 minutes. Serves 4.

Serve each immediately with ⅓ cup cooked brown rice, 6 to 8 steamed asparagus spears and a slice of garlic bread with ½ teaspoon reduced-fat margarine.

Exchanges: 3 meats, 2 breads, 1 vegetable, 1 fruit, ½ fat

~~~~~~

Chicken Linguine

- 12 oz. cooked boneless chicken breasts, cut into bite-sized pieces
- 4 oz. dry linguini
- 1 tbsp. reduced-fat margarine
- ½ c. red bell peppers, chopped
- ½ c. onion, chopped
- 1 c. mushrooms, sliced
- 1 oz. reduced-fat Jarlsberg or Swiss cheese, shredded
- 2 garlic cloves, minced
- 1 tsp. dry leaf oregano, crushed
- 2 c. broccoli florets
- ½ c. evaporated nonfat milk
- ½ c. scallions, sliced
- ¼ c. fresh Parmesan cheese, shredded

Cook pasta according to package directions (omitting salt and fat). Drain and set aside. Melt margarine in large nonstick skillet and sauté peppers, onion, garlic, mushrooms and oregano. Cook for 5 minutes, stirring occasionally. Add chicken and remaining ingredients; then cook until cheese is melted, stirring constantly. Add linguini and mix well. Serves 4. (Refrigerate leftovers immediately for a great cold pasta salad.)

Serve with 1 cup fruit salad mixed with 1 tablespoon low-fat vanilla yogurt.

Exchanges: 3 meats, 2 breads, 2 vegetables, 1 fruit, ¼ milk, ½ fat

~~~~~~

Salmon Cakes

- 1 15½-oz. can red salmon, drained
- 2 tsp. onion, minced
- 1 2-oz. jar diced pimentos
- 6 saltines, crushed
- 3 tbsp. reduced-fat Miracle Whip
- 1 tsp. lemon juice
- 3 drops Tabasco sauce
- Butter-flavored nonstick cooking spray

Remove skin and large bones from fish. Combine remaining ingredients in medium mixing bowl, mashing any remaining bones with a fork. Shape mixture into 4 patties. Coat medium skillet with nonstick cooking spray. Cook salmon cakes over medium-high heat until lightly browned on each side.

Serve with ½ cup garlic mashed potatoes, 1 cup Creole green beans and a medium piece of fruit.

Exchanges: 1½ meats, 2 breads, 1 vegetable, 1 fruit, 1 fat

~~~~~~

Spicy Chicken Stir-Fry Fettuccine

- 6 oz. fettuccine noodles
- 2 tbsp. olive oil
- 3 garlic cloves, minced
- ¾ tsp. black pepper
- 1 lb. chicken tenders
- ½ tsp. salt
- 8 oz. mushrooms, sliced
- 1 10-oz. can Rotel tomatoes
- ¼ c. fresh Parmesan cheese, grated

Cook pasta according to package directions (omitting salt and fat). Drain well and leave cooked pasta in pot. Mix oil, garlic and pepper in medium bowl; add chicken and toss to coat. Heat large nonstick skillet over medium heat and stir-fry chicken 2 to 3 minutes. Remove from skillet with slotted spoon and sprinkle with salt. Add mushrooms to skillet and stir-fry for 3 minutes. Add tomatoes and cooked chicken, stir well; then pour mixture into pot of pasta. Heat if needed. Add Parmesan and toss well. Serves 4.

Serve each with 1 cup oven-roasted vegetables.

Exchanges: 3 meats, 2 breads, 1½ vegetable, 1 fat

~~~~~~

Grecian Skillet Steaks

- 2 8-oz. lean strip loin steaks, about 1-inch thick
- 1½ tsp. dried leaf oregano, crushed
- 1 tsp. dried leaf basil, crushed
- ½ tsp. salt
- ¼ tsp. black pepper
- 1 tbsp. olive oil
- 3 garlic cloves, minced
- 2 tbsp. feta cheese, crumbled
- 1 tbsp. fresh lemon juice
- 1 tbsp. ripe olives, chopped

Sprinkle both sides of steaks with herbs and seasonings. Heat oil on medium in large skillet. Add garlic and sauté for 1 minute. Add steaks and cook 5 minutes on each side for medium-rare (longer for well-done). Remove from heat and sprinkle with cheese, lemon juice and olives. Cut each steak in half before serving. Serves 4.

Serve each with ½ cup roasted potatoes, 1 cup marinated green beans, a 1-ounce dinner roll and 1 small orange.

Exchanges: 3 meats, 2 breads, 1 vegetable, 1 fruit, 1 fat

~~~~~~

Taco Beef and Pasta

- 4 oz. rotini pasta, uncooked
- 1 lb. round tip steak, about 1-inch thick
- 1 pkg. taco seasoning mix
- 1 tbsp. fresh cilantro, chopped
- 3 garlic cloves, crushed
- 1 tbsp. olive oil
- 2 c. chunky commercial salsa
- 1 15-oz. can black beans, rinsed and drained
- ½ c. water

Cook pasta according to package directions (omitting fat). Cut steak into ¼-inch-thick strips. Combine beef and seasonings; toss to coat. Heat skillet; then sauté half of steak strips over high heat 1 to 2 minutes, or until no longer pink. Remove from skillet with a slotted spoon; set aside. Sauté remaining half in same manner. Add pasta, salsa, beans and water to pan; cook 4 to 5 minutes over medium heat. Combine with beef in serving bowl and garnish as desired. Serves 4.

Serve each with salad of cucumbers and peppers, tossed with reduced-fat dressing and 1 kiwi.

Exchanges: 3 meats, 2½ breads, 1½ vegetable, 1 fruit, 1 fat

~~~~~~

Asparagus Chicken

- ½ lb. chicken tenders
- 2 10-oz. pkg. frozen asparagus, thawed
- 1 10¾-oz. can reduced-fat cream of mushroom soup
- ½ c. reduced-fat mayonnaise
- Butter-flavored nonstick cooking spray
- 1 tbsp. lemon juice
- Dash cayenne pepper
- ¾ c. 3-oz. reduced-fat cheddar cheese, shredded
- ¼ c. seasoned bread crumbs

Preheat oven to 375° F. Coat 8x8-inch baking dish and large skillet each with nonstick cooking spray. Sauté ½ of chicken in skillet 1 to 2 minutes; remove and repeat with remaining chicken. Place asparagus in bottom of baking dish. Arrange chicken over asparagus. Combine soup, mayonnaise, lemon juice and pepper in medium bowl. Pour into skillet and heat until bubbly, stirring constantly. Pour over chicken. Top with cheese and bake for 15 minutes, covered. Remove cover and sprinkle with bread crumbs; then bake 10 more minutes. Serves 4.

Serve with ½ cup cooked rice and 1 small apple.

Exchanges: 3 meats, 2 breads, 1 vegetable, 1 fruit, ½ fat

~~~~~~

Chicken Florentine

- 2 tsp. reduced-fat margarine
- 4 3-oz. boneless, skinless chicken breasts
- 1 10¾-oz. can condensed reduced-fat cream of chicken soup, undiluted
- 2 oz. part-skim mozzarella cheese, shredded
- ⅛ tsp. ground nutmeg
- ⅛ tsp. ground black pepper
- 2 10-oz. pkg. frozen chopped spinach
- 2 tbsp. fresh Parmesan cheese, grated

Preheat oven to 350° F. Melt margarine in large nonstick skillet over medium heat. Sauté chicken breasts 3 to 4 minutes on each side or until browned well. Combine soup, mozzarella and seasonings in medium saucepan. Cook over medium heat until cheese is melted. Line bottom of 13x9-inch baking dish with spinach. Top with chicken in a single layer. Pour cheese sauce evenly over the top; sprinkle with Parmesan cheese and bake for 12-15 minutes. Serves 4.

Serve each with ⅓ cup brown rice, 1 cup steamed cauliflower, a 1-ounce dinner roll and a banana.

Exchanges: 3 meats, 2 breads, 2 vegetables, 1 fruit, 1 fat

~~~~~~

Swiss-Style Chicken

- 3 3-oz. boneless, skinless chicken breasts, cut into 16 strips
- ¾ c. reduced-fat Swiss cheese shredded
- 2 tsp. reduced-fat margarine
- 1 garlic clove, minced
- 1 tsp. Italian seasoning
- 1 c. mushrooms, sliced
- 1 15-oz. can chunky tomato sauce
- 1 tbsp. all-purpose flour
- Butter-flavored nonstick cooking spray
- 2 tsp. sugar

Preheat oven to 350° F. Place chicken in 8x8-inch baking dish coated with nonstick cooking spray. Sprinkle chicken with cheese. Heat margarine in small skillet and sauté garlic 1 minute. Add mushrooms and sauté 2 to 3 minutes, or until tender. Combine tomato sauce, Italian seasoning, flour, sugar and mushrooms in small bowl; mix well and pour over cheese-topped chicken. Bake uncovered for 30 to 35 minutes. Serves 4.

Served with ½ cup cooked rice and 1 cup steamed broccoli.
Exchanges: 3 meats, 1½ breads, 1½ vegetables, 1 fat

Conversion Chart
Equivalent Imperial and Metric Measurements

Liquid Measures

Fluid Ounces	U.S.	Imperial	Milliliters
	1 teaspoon	1 teaspoon	5
1/4	2 teaspoons	1 dessert spoon	7
1/2	1 tablespoon	1 tablespoon	15
1	2 tablespoons	2 tablespoons	28
2	1/4 cup	4 tablespoons	56
4	1/2 cup or 1/4 pint		110
5		1/4 pint or 1 gill	140
6	3/4 cup		170
8	1 cup or 1/2 pint		225
9			250 or 1/4 liter
10	1 1/4 cups	1/2 pint	280
12	1 1/2 cups or 3/4 pint		340
15		3/4 pint	420
16	2 cups or 1 pint		450
18	2 1/4 cups		500 or 1/2 liter
20	2 1/2 cups	1 pint	560
24	3 cups or 1 1/2 pints		675
25		1 1/4	700
30	3 3/4 cups	1 1/2 pints	840
32	4 cups		900
36	4 1/2 cups		1000 or 1 liter
40	5 cups	2 pints or 1 quart	1120
48	6 cups or 3 pints		1350
50		2 1/2 pints	1400

Solid Measures

U.S. and Imperial Measures		Metric Measures	
Ounces	Pounds	Grams	Kilos
1		28	
2		56	
3½		100	
4	¼	112	
5		140	
6		168	
8	½	225	
9		250	¼
12	¾	340	
16	1	450	
18		500	½
20	1¼	560	
24		675	
27		750	¾
32	2	900	
36	2¼	1000	1
40	2½	1100	
48	3	1350	
54		1500	1½
64	4	1800	
72	4½	2000	2
80	5	2250	2¼
100	6	2800	2¾

Oven Temperature Equivalents

Fahrenheit	Celsius	Gas Mark	Description
225	110	¼	Cool
250	130	½	
275	140	1	Very Slow
300	150	2	
325	170	3	Slow
350	180	4	Moderate
375	190	5	
400	200	6	Moderately Hot
425	220	7	Fairly Hot
450	230	8	Hot
475	240	9	Very Hot
500	250	10	Extremely Hot

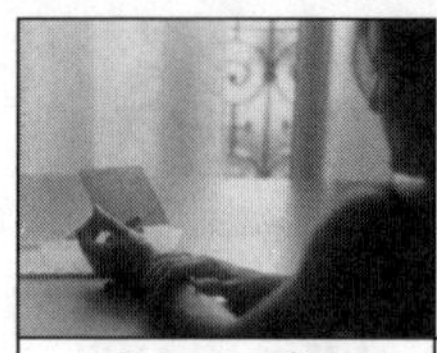

Pressing On
to the Prize

LEADER'S DISCUSSION GUIDE

Week One: Forgetting the Past

1. After reading Philippians 3:13-14, discuss: What do we mean by forgetting the past? Do we literally forget negative experiences?

   After responses, explain that we forget the past when we turn memories into reminders of God's grace, refusing to allow the past to control us, refocusing on what God is doing now.

2. **Before the meeting,** enlist a volunteer to give a testimony of how God helped him or her to forgive a person or circumstance from the past. Lead the group to identify some steps in moving toward forgiveness. Emphasize that for significant hurts forgiveness will be a process. Beware of getting too intimate too soon with this discussion so that members will not be overwhelmed in this first session.

3. Form groups of three or four. Instruct groups to list some practical evidences that indicate a person has (*a*) forgiven and (*b*) forgotten a past hurt. Allow five minutes for discussion. Have one reporter from each small group share their group's list with the large group.

4. The week's emphasis was on not allowing negative experiences from the past to prevent us from pressing on to spiritual victories in the present and future. It also focused on using past skills for new adventures. Invite one or more persons in each small group to take a couple of minutes to share how a person or event from their past has been used by God to positively influence their Christian life and service in the present.

5. Ask volunteers to share other helpful insights that they learned from this week's Bible study.

6. In the past some group members may have had difficulty with health issues. Ask members how past experience with their health and physical well-being affects how they approach this new opportunity in the First Place program. Point out that the past does not have to dictate the future. This week's Bible study shows how members can leave behind the effects of the past.

7. Referring to the Days 6 and 7 Reflections, discuss some of the methods they can use to memorize Scripture. Give examples of how memorizing Scripture can be beneficial in prayer. (Refer to the *Member's Guide*, pages 23 to 25, for additional suggestions.)

8. Ask group members to close their eyes and silently pray this week's verse. Ask them to reflect on how their participation in the First Place program offers them the opportunity to leave all past failures behind them. Close this meditation time by praising God for His partnership with us in forgetting the past.

Week Two: Straining Toward the Future

1. Ask three volunteers to recite Hebrews 11:8 from memory. Ask for volunteers who can quote both last week's and this week's verses from memory.

2. Have volunteers respond to the emphasis on Abraham and his trust in God's promises of an unknown land, inheritance and innumerable descendants. Encourage them to explain why it is important to obey God even when they are not sure how all the details will turn out.

3. Form two equal-sized groups. Instruct each group to discuss how following the First Place program can be like taking a journey into an unknown land.

4. Instruct the groups to review the possible emotional responses of Sarah. Instruct them to formulate a statement that explains how we are to deal with our conflicting feelings when we sense God is calling us to embark on a new adventure for Him. Have each group share with the other group.

5. Summarize Abraham's experiences by discussing: What kept Abraham going on his lifelong journey of faith?

6. In the same two groups, instruct one group to share their response to the vision in Isaiah 6:1-8. Ask the other group to share their responses to John's vision in Revelation 5:11-14. Then have members in each group report how their own reverence and worship of God was increased by the vision they examined.

7. With the whole group, ask members to recall how God used Boaz and Naomi in Ruth's life. Invite volunteers to share how God has used significant individuals in their lives. Remind them that they should thank God for these special people and express their thanks to these people personally if at all possible.

8. Invite a volunteer to read Jeremiah 29:11 aloud. Discuss: What assurance does this verse offer to us? Allow for two or three group responses.

9. Ask if any members tried any of the memorization methods discussed last week to memorize their verse for this week.

10. Close by praying for the faithfulness of the group members, and use Jeremiah 29:11 as a prayer Scripture.

Week Three: Pressing On in the Present

1. Ask three volunteers to quote Mark 4:19, this week's memory verse. Ask if anyone can quote all three verses for this session. Discuss how any of the three threats Jesus mentioned—worries, wealth, desire for other things—could be a stumbling block to pressing on in the present.

2. Form four small groups. Assign one of the following characters discussed in this week's study to each group: Bartimaeus, the man by the pool, the paralytic man and David. Discuss: What new insights gained from this character were particularly applicable to pressing on in the present? Allow time for each group to report to the whole group.

3. Referring to Day 2: Throwing Away Excuses, invite members to share in their small groups how they have already experienced spiritual victory that is helping them overcome the excuse "I have no one to help me" (John 5:7).

4. Ask members to review Ephesians 6:10-18, the full armor of God. Write the six pieces of this armor on a white board or newsprint as members call them out. Give members an opportunity to identify which pieces of armor they are asking God to allow them to use more effectively.

5. Call attention to Day 5: Fighting the Giants. Ask members to identify some of the giants they have already overcome and other giants they still have to overcome in their lives. Remind them that the temptation to eat improperly or not to take care of their bodies is like a giant to be overcome.

6. Form two groups. Assign one group the question: How do you overcome the hurt of negative things others might say to you? Assign the other group the question: How can you pick yourself up when you have experienced failure? After a few minutes of discussion, ask the groups to share their answers.

7. Invite group members to pray silently for themselves and for other group members. After a moment of silent prayer, lead the group in a prayer for strength to meet the challenges they must face as they press on. Use this week's Scripture in your prayer.

Week Four: Claiming My Calling in Christ

1. Recite Colossians 3:14, the memory verse for the week, in unison. Invite members to relate it to Philippians 3:14, this study's theme verse. Discuss: How is your participation in First Place a way of putting on or expressing love for yourself, your family and God, and also pressing on to claim the prize God has for you?

2. Discuss how Christlikeness includes physical fitness and health. Lead the group in conversational prayer, allowing several members to verbally express their goal of achieving balance in every area of life as a way of honoring Christ.

3. Read Psalm 23 in unison. Discuss ways this psalm can be related to their journey in First Place. Discuss: How can the process of becoming healthy and fit feel like being in the valley of the shadow of death? Remind the group that God promises His sufficiency.

4. Read Hebrews 12:11. Remind members that this verse promises a harvest of righteousness for those who will endure the painful training of discipline. Read the stories of Kathy and Angela and Steve and Chuck on page 54. Discuss the attitudes of these four people. Discuss: Which ones are likely to benefit most from their involvement in the First Place program?

5. Write the six Scripture references used in the matching exercise on page 56. Invite volunteers to give the answer for each along with some brief personal feedback on what these verses mean for daily living.

6. Call attention to the activity in which participants wrote portions of Philippians 2:1-5 in their own words. Ask group members to volunteer to share what they wrote.

7. Have members form pairs. Ask each pair to discuss how the qualities described in Ephesians 4:1-4 can help them live lives worthy of their calling.

8. Invite pairs to pray together.

Week Five: Running for the Prize

1. Invite volunteers to quote the five memory verses of this study.
2. Discuss the emphasis for this week: How does the pursuit of spiritual character development help us overcome materialism (see 1 Timothy 5:10) and focus our attention on the prize God has for us?
3. Discuss: How can running for the prize cause us to give greater attention to what we are running toward than what we are running from? Remind them that the prize is intimate fellowship with God.
4. Ask several volunteers to share their responses to the activity on page 62 in which they described how God used one of the listed motivators to inspire victory in the Christian life. Affirm any spiritual victories shared by members so all may be encouraged. Discuss: What are additional motivators for spiritual victories other than those suggested in the study?
5. Have someone read Matthew 22:30-31. Remind the group that righteousness means living a balanced life. These verses reflect the balance God intended for our lives. Ask the group to discuss how we can love God with our total being and give examples of how we can demonstrate loving our neighbor as we love ourselves.
6. Form small groups of three or four. Instruct each small group to review the matching activity on page 67. Then have each group discuss practical examples of how we are justified by faith, shielded by faith and live by faith. Have each group share its work with the whole group.
7. Write the following sentence on the board: "We demonstrate the presence of God in our lives by treating others the way God has treated us." Discuss the statement. Point out that how we treat others greatly affects how closely we can relate to God. Read 1 John 4:20 to emphasize the point.
8. Ask one or more volunteers to report how they responded to the characteristics of the love of Jesus given on page 70. Lead members to understand that God must change our perspective to move us from harshness to gentleness. Remind them that encouragement is one of the commitments of First Place.
9. Close in prayer. Ask God for an eagerness for the race of Christian living and a focus on the prize of intimate fellowship with Him.

Week Six: Training for the Race

1. Ask three volunteers to recite 1 Corinthians 9:24. Ask a volunteer to quote memory verses from previous weeks. Point out that Paul believed that running is for winning—not merely exercising! Winning means receiving the reward you are seeking. Ask for a few brief testimonies of how the First Place program has already been a rewarding experience.

2. Discuss: Why is spiritual training so important if someone is already saved and going to heaven?

3. Form small groups of three or four. Referring to Hebrews 12:1-2, remind members that in order to run to win, believers must not lose their focus or quit their course. Instruct the small groups to share what helps them keep their focus on Jesus. After several minutes for sharing, read Galatians 6:9-10. Remind members that victory is promised to those who do not grow weary and give up. Have them share with their small groups what keeps them from giving up.

4. In the small groups ask them to share their responses to the Bible study activity about the work of the Holy Spirit (p. 81). Invite them to discuss the importance of the teaching, guiding and empowering work of the Holy Spirit in their lives. Have them discuss how the Roy Riegels story relates to their spiritual race. After several minutes, ask them to discuss the importance of the Holy Spirit's role in helping us aim for the goal in Christian living.

5. Ask volunteers to share what they checked as evidences of a Spirit-filled life (p. 82). Invite members to share what being filled with the Spirit means to them.

6. Ask volunteers to share how participating in the First Place program demonstrates that their bodies truly are the temples of the Holy Spirit.

7. Lead in a time of silent prayer for the Holy Spirit's guidance to keep their focus on the prize of fellowship with God.

Week Seven: Receiving an Everlasting Crown

1. Ask a volunteer to recite 1 Peter 5:4. Discuss what the crown of glory from this verse refers to (see 1 Corinthians 9:25).

2. Invite members to identify the major differences between the two different crowns of David and Absalom. Write these differences on the board. Lead the group to reflect on how knowing God's calling for our

lives helps us stay focused even in hard times. Call for testimonies about God's provision in times of difficulty. Remind members of God's help in keeping the nine commitments of First Place.

3. Form small groups of three or four. Assign the small groups one or more of the crowns studied this week. Provide construction paper, felt-tip pens, staplers or transparent tape and scissors for each small group to make and label their crown(s). Have volunteers from each small group wear their group's crowns when they report on the meaning of that crown.

4. Reconvene the whole group. Remind members that the everlasting crown symbolizes the prize of intimate fellowship with God. Help them understand that each crown is a result of their fellowship. Invite volunteers to describe how fellowship with God has been enhanced for them by daily quiet time.

5. Have a volunteer read 2 Timothy 4:6-8 and review the three actions Paul had accomplished in his life. Help members apply each of these concepts to the First Place program. Discuss the implications of not having to earn our reward with good works but having it given as a sign of intimate relationship with God. Have a volunteer read Matthew 5:6, in which Jesus promised that God will completely satisfy those who wholeheartedly pursue righteousness.

6. Ask volunteers to share what they wrote or drew about worshiping in the presence of God someday (p. 93).

7. Close in prayer, thanking God for the everlasting crown we can receive from Him. Ask Him to remind us daily how this crown has greater value than any other treasure.

Week Eight: Removing Every Obstacle

1. Invite volunteers to recite Hebrews 12:1 from memory. Remind members that every spiritual runner has obstacles to overcome. Ask volunteers to share what obstacles they have overcome to remain active in First Place.

2. Discuss why God allows us to have obstacles when we are trying to have intimate fellowship with Him. Lead the group to understand that we are often strengthened as we experience God's faithfulness in confronting obstacles.

3. Form small groups of three or four. Assign each small group one or more of the obstacles from this week's study. Instruct each group to

draw a picture on a large sheet of newsprint to symbolize how they see their obstacle(s) manifesting itself (themselves) today. Provide felt-tip pens and paper for each group.

4. Have groups report to the whole group on the following: (*a*) read a key verse for each obstacle found in the study materials and (*b*) report what new insights members learned about their obstacle(s) and how it (they) could be overcome. Mount the papers around the room for all participants to see.

5. Reconvene the whole group. Remind members that each obstacle in our path has a purpose. God wants to use them as motivators and not barriers in developing intimate fellowship with Him. Have volunteers share how God has used the removal of one of the obstacles in their lives to bring them closer to Him.

6. Discuss the obstacle of possessiveness. Review how the perspective of stewardship rather than ownership applies to self, people and things. Have a volunteer share how victory over possessiveness has made a positive difference in a significant relationship with another person.

7. Have someone read 2 Thessalonians 3:6-13. Point out how Paul warned that self-indulgence can produce a lifestyle of idleness, gossip and nosiness. Discuss how this statement is true in our culture today. Discuss: What can churches do to more effectively overcome this problem?

8. Discuss how prayer and Scripture memory can help overcome the obstacles we face every day. Discuss obstacles to their Scripture memorization and how to overcome them.

9. Close in prayer, thanking God for His power to overcome obstacles that seem insurmountable to us.

Week Nine: Looking to Jesus

1. Have volunteers recite Hebrews 12:2 from memory. Remind members the purpose of this week's study was to focus on Jesus as we press on to the prize of intimate fellowship with God. Invite volunteers to share how looking to Jesus has encouraged them to stay with the disciplines of the First Place program.

2. Discuss why it is important to keep looking to Jesus every step of the way in the believer's spiritual journey. Ask a volunteer to read Hebrews 12:3. Point out that without the continual example of seeing Christ as our fellow struggler and sojourner, even the most mature believer can grow weary and lose heart.

3. Form small groups of three or four. Assign each small group one or more of the seven roles of Jesus from this week's study. Have each group write a paragraph summarizing how they see Jesus in the role(s) assigned to them. Some groups may want to draw on a sheet of newsprint a picture of Jesus in the role(s) assigned to them. Or some may choose to act out a brief skit to illustrate how they see Jesus functioning in the role(s). Provide felt-tip pens and paper for each group.

4. As groups share their summaries, ask them to include: (*a*) a key verse for each role from the day's study and (*b*) new insights about Jesus that they learned from the study.

5. Reconvene the whole group. Point out that each role of Jesus is revealed to us for a purpose. God wants us to have concrete mental images of His Son to carry in our hearts in order to produce a more intimate fellowship between God the Father and us.

6. Invite volunteers to share a miracle they have asked God to work in their lives or one they have seen God perform recently.

7. Focus attention on the final image of Jesus sitting on His throne. Discuss: How does seeing yourself sitting on Jesus' throne with Him give you renewed motivation for the daily struggles you face? Encourage testimonies of how the First Place program has helped them feel supported by other Christians in facing their struggles.

8. Ask volunteers to share how praying God's Word with the use of Scriptures has enhanced their prayer life.

9. Thank God for the pictures He gives us of the many roles Jesus has in every aspect of our lives.

Week Ten: God's Love for You

1. Invite volunteers to recite all 10 memory verses. Discuss briefly the methods members used to aid in Scripture memory.

2. Recite Hebrews 12:15 in unison. Remind members that the purpose of this week's study was to concentrate on seven avenues for accepting the grace of God so that a root of bitterness does not defile God's grace. Ask to share how a focus on grace has enabled them to complete the past 10 weeks of the First Place program.

3. Invite members to share why it is important to keep focusing on God's grace as we press on to the prize of intimate fellowship with God. Have

someone recite Philippians 3:14 from memory. This verse is the theme memory verse for this study.

4. Form small groups of three or four. Assign the small groups one or more of the seven avenues for accepting the grace of God. Have each group write a summary of how the avenue(s) assigned to them can help believers grow in intimate relationship with God. Or some may choose to act out a brief skit or draw a picture. Provide felt-tip pens and paper for each group.

5. As groups report, ask them to include in their presentations: (*a*) a key verse for each avenue and (*b*) new insights about applying grace that they learned from the study.

6. Reconvene the whole group for sharing. Remind members that these avenues for practicing God's grace are given to us for a purpose. God wants us to have in mind specific ways of remaining open to His grace in daily living.

7. Review the story in Genesis 33:8-17 where Esau is an example of practicing forgiveness. Invite members to share how they have seen their health and happiness improved by being able to forgive someone.

8. Ask volunteers to share about a time in which they have had their own spirits lifted by thanking God for His blessings.

9. Close by thanking members for their participation in this study. Lead in prayer, thanking God for the way the First Place program has helped individuals become grace-filled believers. Give a word of encouragement to participants as they leave.

PERSONAL WEIGHT RECORD

Week	Weight	+ or -	Goal This Session	Pounds to Goal
1				
2				
3				
4				
5				
6				
7				
8				
9				
10				
11				
12				
13				
Final				

Beginning Measurements

Waist_____ Hips_____ Thighs_____ Chest_____

Ending Measurements

Waist_____ Hips_____ Thighs_____ Chest_____

Commitment Records

How to Fill Out a Commitment Record

The Commitment Record (CR) is an aid for you in keeping track of your accomplishments. Begin a new CR on the morning of the day your class meets. This ensures that your CR is complete before your next meeting. Turn in the CR weekly to your leader.

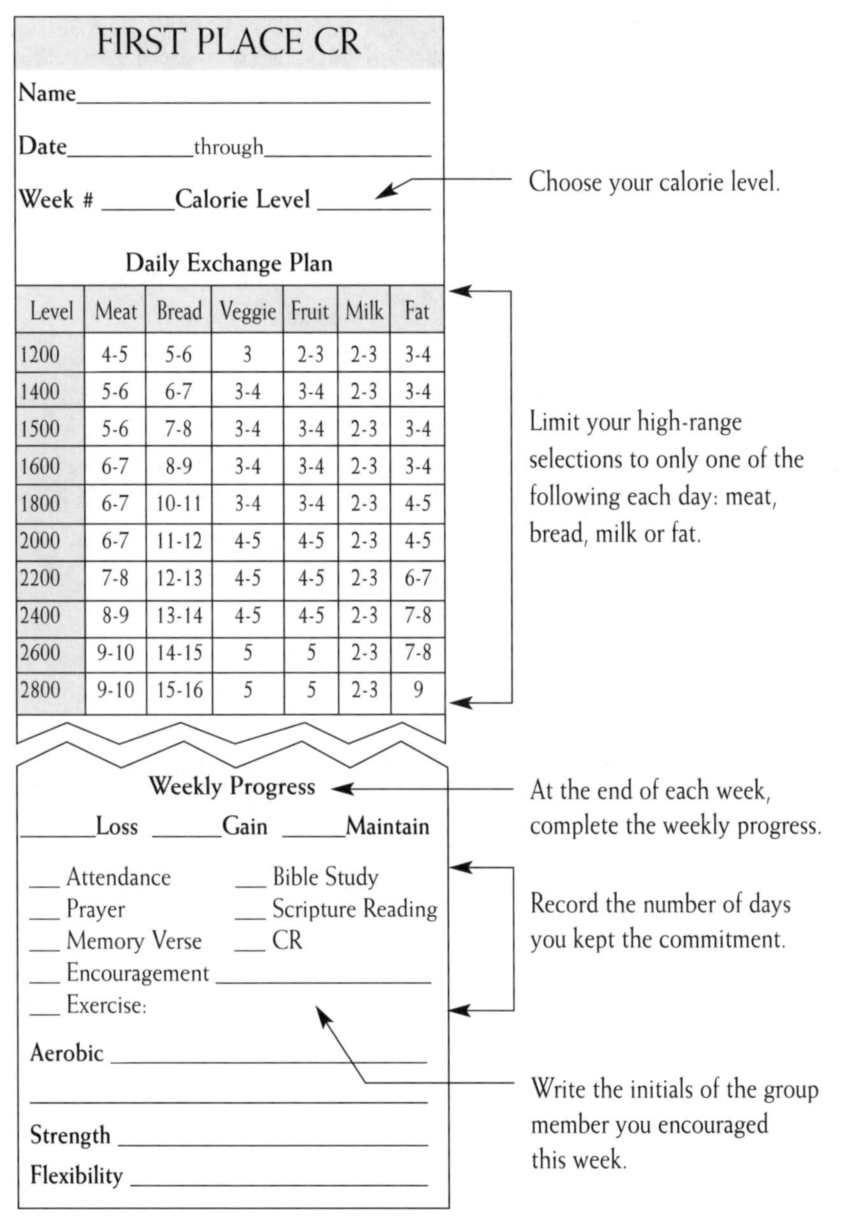

FIRST PLACE CR

Name________________________

Date__________through______________

Week # ______Calorie Level __________

Daily Exchange Plan

Level	Meat	Bread	Veggie	Fruit	Milk	Fat
1200	4-5	5-6	3	2-3	2-3	3-4
1400	5-6	6-7	3-4	3-4	2-3	3-4
1500	5-6	7-8	3-4	3-4	2-3	3-4
1600	6-7	8-9	3-4	3-4	2-3	3-4
1800	6-7	10-11	3-4	3-4	2-3	4-5
2000	6-7	11-12	4-5	4-5	2-3	4-5
2200	7-8	12-13	4-5	4-5	2-3	6-7
2400	8-9	13-14	4-5	4-5	2-3	7-8
2600	9-10	14-15	5	5	2-3	7-8
2800	9-10	15-16	5	5	2-3	9

Weekly Progress

______Loss ______Gain ______Maintain

___ Attendance ___ Bible Study
___ Prayer ___ Scripture Reading
___ Memory Verse ___ CR
___ Encouragement ______________
___ Exercise:

Aerobic ______________________

____

Strength _____________________

Flexibility ___________________

DAY 7: Date ____________

Morning ____________

Midday ____________

Evening ____________

Snacks ____________

___ Meat ______ ☐ Prayer
___ Bread ______ ☐ Bible Study
___ Vegetable ______ ☐ Scripture Reading
___ Fruit ______ ☐ Memory Verse
___ Milk ______ ☐ Encouragement
___ Fat ______ ☐ Water______

Exercise:

Aerobic ____________

Strength ____________

Flexibility ____________

List the foods you have eaten. On this condensed CR it is not necessary to exchange each food choice. It will be the responsibility of each member that the tally marks you list below are accurate regarding each food choice. If you are unsure of an exchange, check the Live-It section of your copy of the *Member's Guide*.

List the daily food exchange choices to the left of the food groups.

Use tally marks for the actual food and water consumed.

Check off commitments completed. Use tally marks to record each 8-oz. serving of water.

List type and duration of exercise.

DAY 5: Date ____

Morning ____

Midday ____

Evening ____

Snacks ____

___ **Meat** ____ ☐ Prayer
___ **Bread** ____ ☐ Bible Study
___ **Vegetable** ____ ☐ Scripture Reading
___ **Fruit** ____ ☐ Memory Verse
___ **Milk** ____ ☐ Encouragement
___ **Fat** ____ Water ____

Exercise
Aerobic ____

Strength ____
Flexibility ____

DAY 6: Date ____

Morning ____

Midday ____

Evening ____

Snacks ____

___ **Meat** ____ ☐ Prayer
___ **Bread** ____ ☐ Bible Study
___ **Vegetable** ____ ☐ Scripture Reading
___ **Fruit** ____ ☐ Memory Verse
___ **Milk** ____ ☐ Encouragement
___ **Fat** ____ Water ____

Exercise
Aerobic ____

Strength ____
Flexibility ____

DAY 7: Date ____

Morning ____

Midday ____

Evening ____

Snacks ____

___ **Meat** ____ ☐ Prayer
___ **Bread** ____ ☐ Bible Study
___ **Vegetable** ____ ☐ Scripture Reading
___ **Fruit** ____ ☐ Memory Verse
___ **Milk** ____ ☐ Encouragement
___ **Fat** ____ Water ____

Exercise
Aerobic ____

Strength ____
Flexibility ____

FIRST PLACE CR

Name ____
Date ____ through ____
Week # ____ **Calorie Level** ____

Daily Exchange Plan

Level	Meat	Bread	Veggie	Fruit	Milk	Fat
1200	4-5	5-6	3	2-3	2-3	3-4
1400	5-6	6-7	3-4	3-4	2-3	3-4
1500	5-6	7-8	3-4	3-4	2-3	3-4
1600	6-7	8-9	3-4	3-4	2-3	3-4
1800	6-7	10-11	3-4	3-4	2-3	4-5
2000	6-7	11-12	4-5	4-5	2-3	4-5
2200	7-8	12-13	4-5	4-5	2-3	6-7
2400	8-9	13-14	4-5	4-5	2-3	7-8
2600	9-10	14-15	5	5	2-3	7-8
2800	9-10	15-16	5	5	2-3	9

You may always choose the high range of vegetables and fruits. Limit your high range selections to only one of the following: meat, bread, milk or fat.

Weekly Progress

____ Loss ____ Gain ____ Maintain

___ Attendance ___ Bible Study
___ Prayer ___ Scripture Reading
___ Memory Verse ___ CR
___ Encouragement: ____
___ Exercise
Aerobic ____

Strength ____
Flexibility ____

DAY 1: Date ______

Morning ______

Midday ______

Evening ______

Snacks ______

___ **Meat** ______ ☐ Prayer
___ **Bread** ______ ☐ Bible Study
___ **Vegetable** ______ ☐ Scripture Reading
___ **Fruit** ______ ☐ Memory Verse
___ **Milk** ______ ☐ Encouragement
___ **Fat** ______ Water ______

Exercise
Aerobic ______
Strength ______
Flexibility ______

DAY 2: Date ______

Morning ______

Midday ______

Evening ______

Snacks ______

___ **Meat** ______ ☐ Prayer
___ **Bread** ______ ☐ Bible Study
___ **Vegetable** ______ ☐ Scripture Reading
___ **Fruit** ______ ☐ Memory Verse
___ **Milk** ______ ☐ Encouragement
___ **Fat** ______ Water ______

Exercise
Aerobic ______
Strength ______
Flexibility ______

DAY 3: Date ______

Morning ______

Midday ______

Evening ______

Snacks ______

___ **Meat** ______ ☐ Prayer
___ **Bread** ______ ☐ Bible Study
___ **Vegetable** ______ ☐ Scripture Reading
___ **Fruit** ______ ☐ Memory Verse
___ **Milk** ______ ☐ Encouragement
___ **Fat** ______ Water ______

Exercise
Aerobic ______
Strength ______
Flexibility ______

DAY 4: Date ______

Morning ______

Midday ______

Evening ______

Snacks ______

___ **Meat** ______ ☐ Prayer
___ **Bread** ______ ☐ Bible Study
___ **Vegetable** ______ ☐ Scripture Reading
___ **Fruit** ______ ☐ Memory Verse
___ **Milk** ______ ☐ Encouragement
___ **Fat** ______ Water ______

Exercise
Aerobic ______
Strength ______
Flexibility ______

DAY 5: Date ____________

Morning ____________

____

____

Midday ____________

____

____

Evening ____________

____

____

Snacks ____________

____

____

___ **Meat** ________ ☐ Prayer
___ **Bread** ________ ☐ Bible Study
___ **Vegetable** _____ ☐ Scripture Reading
___ **Fruit** ________ ☐ Memory Verse
___ **Milk** ________ ☐ Encouragement
___ **Fat** ________ Water ________

Exercise
Aerobic ____________

____

Strength ____________
Flexibility ____________

DAY 6: Date ____________

Morning ____________

____

____

Midday ____________

____

____

Evening ____________

____

____

Snacks ____________

____

____

___ **Meat** ________ ☐ Prayer
___ **Bread** ________ ☐ Bible Study
___ **Vegetable** _____ ☐ Scripture Reading
___ **Fruit** ________ ☐ Memory Verse
___ **Milk** ________ ☐ Encouragement
___ **Fat** ________ Water ________

Exercise
Aerobic ____________

____

Strength ____________
Flexibility ____________

DAY 7: Date ____________

Morning ____________

____

____

Midday ____________

____

____

Evening ____________

____

____

Snacks ____________

____

____

___ **Meat** ________ ☐ Prayer
___ **Bread** ________ ☐ Bible Study
___ **Vegetable** _____ ☐ Scripture Reading
___ **Fruit** ________ ☐ Memory Verse
___ **Milk** ________ ☐ Encouragement
___ **Fat** ________ Water ________

Exercise
Aerobic ____________

____

Strength ____________
Flexibility ____________

FIRST PLACE CR

Name ____________

Date ________ through ________

Week # ______ Calorie Level ________

Daily Exchange Plan

Level	Meat	Bread	Veggie	Fruit	Milk	Fat
1200	4-5	5-6	3	2-3	2-3	3-4
1400	5-6	6-7	3-4	3-4	2-3	3-4
1500	5-6	7-8	3-4	3-4	2-3	3-4
1600	6-7	8-9	3-4	3-4	2-3	3-4
1800	6-7	10-11	3-4	3-4	2-3	4-5
2000	6-7	11-12	4-5	4-5	2-3	4-5
2200	7-8	12-13	4-5	4-5	2-3	6-7
2400	8-9	13-14	4-5	4-5	2-3	7-8
2600	9-10	14-15	5	5	2-3	7-8
2800	9-10	15-16	5	5	2-3	9

You may always choose the high range of vegetables and fruits. Limit your high range selections to only one of the following: meat, bread, milk or fat.

______ Loss ______ Gain ______ Maintain

___ Attendance ___ Bible Study
___ Prayer ___ Scripture Reading
___ Memory Verse ___ CR
___ Encouragement ____________
___ Exercise

Aerobic ____________

____

Strength ____________
Flexibility ____________

DAY 1: Date ________

Morning ________

____

____

Midday ________

____

____

Evening ________

____

____

Snacks ________

____

____

___ **Meat** ________ ☐ Prayer
___ **Bread** ________ ☐ Bible Study
___ **Vegetable** ____ ☐ Scripture Reading
___ **Fruit** ________ ☐ Memory Verse
___ **Milk** ________ ☐ Encouragement
___ **Fat** ________ Water ________

Exercise
Aerobic ________

____

Strength ________
Flexibility ________

DAY 2: Date ________

Morning ________

____

____

Midday ________

____

____

Evening ________

____

____

Snacks ________

____

____

___ **Meat** ________ ☐ Prayer
___ **Bread** ________ ☐ Bible Study
___ **Vegetable** ____ ☐ Scripture Reading
___ **Fruit** ________ ☐ Memory Verse
___ **Milk** ________ ☐ Encouragement
___ **Fat** ________ Water ________

Exercise
Aerobic ________

____

Strength ________
Flexibility ________

DAY 3: Date ________

Morning ________

____

____

Midday ________

____

____

Evening ________

____

____

Snacks ________

____

____

___ **Meat** ________ ☐ Prayer
___ **Bread** ________ ☐ Bible Study
___ **Vegetable** ____ ☐ Scripture Reading
___ **Fruit** ________ ☐ Memory Verse
___ **Milk** ________ ☐ Encouragement
___ **Fat** ________ Water ________

Exercise
Aerobic ________

____

Strength ________
Flexibility ________

DAY 4: Date ________

Morning ________

____

____

Midday ________

____

____

Evening ________

____

____

Snacks ________

____

____

___ **Meat** ________ ☐ Prayer
___ **Bread** ________ ☐ Bible Study
___ **Vegetable** ____ ☐ Scripture Reading
___ **Fruit** ________ ☐ Memory Verse
___ **Milk** ________ ☐ Encouragement
___ **Fat** ________ Water ________

Exercise
Aerobic ________

____

Strength ________
Flexibility ________

DAY 5: Date ____________

Morning ____________

____

____

Midday ____________

____

____

Evening ____________

____

____

Snacks ____________

____

____

___ Meat ______ ☐ Prayer
___ Bread ______ ☐ Bible Study
___ Vegetable ____ ☐ Scripture Reading
___ Fruit ______ ☐ Memory Verse
___ Milk ______ ☐ Encouragement
___ Fat ______ Water ______

Exercise
Aerobic ____________

____

Strength ____________
Flexibility ____________

DAY 6: Date ____________

Morning ____________

____

____

Midday ____________

____

____

Evening ____________

____

____

Snacks ____________

____

____

___ Meat ______ ☐ Prayer
___ Bread ______ ☐ Bible Study
___ Vegetable ____ ☐ Scripture Reading
___ Fruit ______ ☐ Memory Verse
___ Milk ______ ☐ Encouragement
___ Fat ______ Water ______

Exercise
Aerobic ____________

____

Strength ____________
Flexibility ____________

DAY 7: Date ____________

Morning ____________

____

____

Midday ____________

____

____

Evening ____________

____

____

Snacks ____________

____

____

___ Meat ______ ☐ Prayer
___ Bread ______ ☐ Bible Study
___ Vegetable ____ ☐ Scripture Reading
___ Fruit ______ ☐ Memory Verse
___ Milk ______ ☐ Encouragement
___ Fat ______ Water ______

Exercise
Aerobic ____________

____

Strength ____________
Flexibility ____________

FIRST PLACE CR

Name ____________
Date ______ through ______
Week # ______ **Calorie Level** ______

Daily Exchange Plan

Level	Meat	Bread	Veggie	Fruit	Milk	Fat
1200	4-5	5-6	3	2-3	2-3	3-4
1400	5-6	6-7	3-4	3-4	2-3	3-4
1500	5-6	7-8	3-4	3-4	2-3	3-4
1600	6-7	8-9	3-4	3-4	2-3	3-4
1800	6-7	10-11	3-4	3-4	2-3	4-5
2000	6-7	11-12	4-5	4-5	2-3	4-5
2200	7-8	12-13	4-5	4-5	2-3	6-7
2400	8-9	13-14	4-5	4-5	2-3	7-8
2600	9-10	14-15	5	5	2-3	7-8
2800	9-10	15-16	5	5	2-3	9

You may always choose the high range of vegetables and fruits. Limit your high range selections to only one of the following: meat, bread, milk or fat.

_____ Loss _____ Gain _____ Maintain

___ Attendance ___ Bible Study
___ Prayer ___ Scripture Reading
___ Memory Verse ___ CR
___ Encouragement ____________
___ Exercise
Aerobic ____________

____

Strength ____________
Flexibility ____________

DAY 1: Date ____________

Morning ____________

Midday ____________

Evening ____________

Snacks ____________

___ **Meat** ______ ☐ Prayer
___ **Bread** ______ ☐ Bible Study
___ **Vegetable** ____ ☐ Scripture Reading
___ **Fruit** ______ ☐ Memory Verse
___ **Milk** ______ ☐ Encouragement
___ **Fat** ______ Water ______

Exercise
Aerobic ____________
Strength ____________
Flexibility ____________

DAY 2: Date ____________

Morning ____________

Midday ____________

Evening ____________

Snacks ____________

___ **Meat** ______ ☐ Prayer
___ **Bread** ______ ☐ Bible Study
___ **Vegetable** ____ ☐ Scripture Reading
___ **Fruit** ______ ☐ Memory Verse
___ **Milk** ______ ☐ Encouragement
___ **Fat** ______ Water ______

Exercise
Aerobic ____________
Strength ____________
Flexibility ____________

DAY 3: Date ____________

Morning ____________

Midday ____________

Evening ____________

Snacks ____________

___ **Meat** ______ ☐ Prayer
___ **Bread** ______ ☐ Bible Study
___ **Vegetable** ____ ☐ Scripture Reading
___ **Fruit** ______ ☐ Memory Verse
___ **Milk** ______ ☐ Encouragement
___ **Fat** ______ Water ______

Exercise
Aerobic ____________
Strength ____________
Flexibility ____________

DAY 4: Date ____________

Morning ____________

Midday ____________

Evening ____________

Snacks ____________

___ **Meat** ______ ☐ Prayer
___ **Bread** ______ ☐ Bible Study
___ **Vegetable** ____ ☐ Scripture Reading
___ **Fruit** ______ ☐ Memory Verse
___ **Milk** ______ ☐ Encouragement
___ **Fat** ______ Water ______

Exercise
Aerobic ____________
Strength ____________
Flexibility ____________

DAY 5: Date ____________

Morning ____________________

____

____

Midday ____________________

____

____

Evening ____________________

____

____

Snacks ____________________

____

____

___ **Meat** ________ ☐ Prayer
___ **Bread** ________ ☐ Bible Study
___ **Vegetable** ________ ☐ Scripture Reading
___ **Fruit** ________ ☐ Memory Verse
___ **Milk** ________ ☐ Encouragement
___ **Fat** ________ Water ________

Exercise
Aerobic ____________________

____

Strength ____________________
Flexibility ____________________

DAY 6: Date ____________

Morning ____________________

____

____

Midday ____________________

____

____

Evening ____________________

____

____

Snacks ____________________

____

____

___ **Meat** ________ ☐ Prayer
___ **Bread** ________ ☐ Bible Study
___ **Vegetable** ________ ☐ Scripture Reading
___ **Fruit** ________ ☐ Memory Verse
___ **Milk** ________ ☐ Encouragement
___ **Fat** ________ Water ________

Exercise
Aerobic ____________________

____

Strength ____________________
Flexibility ____________________

DAY 7: Date ____________

Morning ____________________

____

____

Midday ____________________

____

____

Evening ____________________

____

____

Snacks ____________________

____

____

___ **Meat** ________ ☐ Prayer
___ **Bread** ________ ☐ Bible Study
___ **Vegetable** ________ ☐ Scripture Reading
___ **Fruit** ________ ☐ Memory Verse
___ **Milk** ________ ☐ Encouragement
___ **Fat** ________ Water ________

Exercise
Aerobic ____________________

____

Strength ____________________
Flexibility ____________________

FIRST PLACE CR

Name ____________________

Date __________ through __________

Week # ______ **Calorie Level** __________

Daily Exchange Plan

Level	Meat	Bread	Veggie	Fruit	Milk	Fat
1200	4-5	5-6	3	2-3	2-3	3-4
1400	5-6	6-7	3-4	3-4	2-3	3-4
1500	5-6	7-8	3-4	3-4	2-3	3-4
1600	6-7	8-9	3-4	3-4	2-3	3-4
1800	6-7	10-11	3-4	3-4	2-3	4-5
2000	6-7	11-12	4-5	4-5	2-3	4-5
2200	7-8	12-13	4-5	4-5	2-3	6-7
2400	8-9	13-14	4-5	4-5	2-3	7-8
2600	9-10	14-15	5	5	2-3	7-8
2800	9-10	15-16	5	5	2-3	9

You may always choose the high range of vegetables and fruits. Limit your high range selections to only one of the following: meat, bread, milk or fat.

______Loss ______Gain ______Maintain

___ Attendance ___ Bible Study
___ Prayer ___ Scripture Reading
___ Memory Verse ___ CR
___ Encouragement ____________
___ Exercise
Aerobic ____________________

____

Strength ____________________
Flexibility ____________________

DAY 1: Date ____

Morning ____

Midday ____

Evening ____

Snacks ____

___ **Meat** ____ ☐ Prayer
___ **Bread** ____ ☐ Bible Study
___ **Vegetable** ____ ☐ Scripture Reading
___ **Fruit** ____ ☐ Memory Verse
___ **Milk** ____ ☐ Encouragement
___ **Fat** ____ Water ____

Exercise
Aerobic ____
Strength ____
Flexibility ____

DAY 2: Date ____

Morning ____

Midday ____

Evening ____

Snacks ____

___ **Meat** ____ ☐ Prayer
___ **Bread** ____ ☐ Bible Study
___ **Vegetable** ____ ☐ Scripture Reading
___ **Fruit** ____ ☐ Memory Verse
___ **Milk** ____ ☐ Encouragement
___ **Fat** ____ Water ____

Exercise
Aerobic ____
Strength ____
Flexibility ____

DAY 3: Date ____

Morning ____

Midday ____

Evening ____

Snacks ____

___ **Meat** ____ ☐ Prayer
___ **Bread** ____ ☐ Bible Study
___ **Vegetable** ____ ☐ Scripture Reading
___ **Fruit** ____ ☐ Memory Verse
___ **Milk** ____ ☐ Encouragement
___ **Fat** ____ Water ____

Exercise
Aerobic ____
Strength ____
Flexibility ____

DAY 4: Date ____

Morning ____

Midday ____

Evening ____

Snacks ____

___ **Meat** ____ ☐ Prayer
___ **Bread** ____ ☐ Bible Study
___ **Vegetable** ____ ☐ Scripture Reading
___ **Fruit** ____ ☐ Memory Verse
___ **Milk** ____ ☐ Encouragement
___ **Fat** ____ Water ____

Exercise
Aerobic ____
Strength ____
Flexibility ____

DAY 5: Date ____________

Morning ____________

Midday ____________

Evening ____________

Snacks ____________

___ **Meat** ______ ☐ Prayer
___ **Bread** ______ ☐ Bible Study
___ **Vegetable** ______ ☐ Scripture Reading
___ **Fruit** ______ ☐ Memory Verse
___ **Milk** ______ ☐ Encouragement
___ **Fat** ______ Water ______

Exercise
Aerobic ____________
Strength ____________
Flexibility ____________

DAY 6: Date ____________

Morning ____________

Midday ____________

Evening ____________

Snacks ____________

___ **Meat** ______ ☐ Prayer
___ **Bread** ______ ☐ Bible Study
___ **Vegetable** ______ ☐ Scripture Reading
___ **Fruit** ______ ☐ Memory Verse
___ **Milk** ______ ☐ Encouragement
___ **Fat** ______ Water ______

Exercise
Aerobic ____________
Strength ____________
Flexibility ____________

DAY 7: Date ____________

Morning ____________

Midday ____________

Evening ____________

Snacks ____________

___ **Meat** ______ ☐ Prayer
___ **Bread** ______ ☐ Bible Study
___ **Vegetable** ______ ☐ Scripture Reading
___ **Fruit** ______ ☐ Memory Verse
___ **Milk** ______ ☐ Encouragement
___ **Fat** ______ Water ______

Exercise
Aerobic ____________
Strength ____________
Flexibility ____________

FIRST PLACE CR

Name ____________
Date ______ through ______
Week # ______ **Calorie Level** ______

Daily Exchange Plan

Level	Meat	Bread	Veggie	Fruit	Milk	Fat
1200	4-5	5-6	3	2-3	2-3	3-4
1400	5-6	6-7	3-4	3-4	2-3	3-4
1500	5-6	7-8	3-4	3-4	2-3	3-4
1600	6-7	8-9	3-4	3-4	2-3	3-4
1800	6-7	10-11	3-4	3-4	2-3	4-5
2000	6-7	11-12	4-5	4-5	2-3	4-5
2200	7-8	12-13	4-5	4-5	2-3	6-7
2400	8-9	13-14	4-5	4-5	2-3	7-8
2600	9-10	14-15	5	5	2-3	7-8
2800	9-10	15-16	5	5	2-3	9

You may always choose the high range of vegetables and fruits. Limit your high range selections to only one of the following: meat, bread, milk or fat.

______ Loss ______ Gain ______ Maintain

___ Attendance ___ Bible Study
___ Prayer ___ Scripture Reading
___ Memory Verse ___ CR
___ Encouragement ____________
___ Exercise

Aerobic ____________
Strength ____________
Flexibility ____________

DAY 1: Date ____________

Morning ____________

Midday ____________

Evening ____________

Snacks ____________

___ **Meat** ______ ☐ Prayer
___ **Bread** ______ ☐ Bible Study
___ **Vegetable** ______ ☐ Scripture Reading
___ **Fruit** ______ ☐ Memory Verse
___ **Milk** ______ ☐ Encouragement
___ **Fat** ______ Water ______

Exercise
Aerobic ____________
Strength ____________
Flexibility ____________

DAY 2: Date ____________

Morning ____________

Midday ____________

Evening ____________

Snacks ____________

___ **Meat** ______ ☐ Prayer
___ **Bread** ______ ☐ Bible Study
___ **Vegetable** ______ ☐ Scripture Reading
___ **Fruit** ______ ☐ Memory Verse
___ **Milk** ______ ☐ Encouragement
___ **Fat** ______ Water ______

Exercise
Aerobic ____________
Strength ____________
Flexibility ____________

DAY 3: Date ____________

Morning ____________

Midday ____________

Evening ____________

Snacks ____________

___ **Meat** ______ ☐ Prayer
___ **Bread** ______ ☐ Bible Study
___ **Vegetable** ______ ☐ Scripture Reading
___ **Fruit** ______ ☐ Memory Verse
___ **Milk** ______ ☐ Encouragement
___ **Fat** ______ Water ______

Exercise
Aerobic ____________
Strength ____________
Flexibility ____________

DAY 4: Date ____________

Morning ____________

Midday ____________

Evening ____________

Snacks ____________

___ **Meat** ______ ☐ Prayer
___ **Bread** ______ ☐ Bible Study
___ **Vegetable** ______ ☐ Scripture Reading
___ **Fruit** ______ ☐ Memory Verse
___ **Milk** ______ ☐ Encouragement
___ **Fat** ______ Water ______

Exercise
Aerobic ____________
Strength ____________
Flexibility ____________

DAY 5: Date ____________

Morning ____________

____

____

Midday ____________

____

____

Evening ____________

____

____

Snacks ____________

____

____

___ **Meat** ________ ☐ Prayer

___ **Bread** ________ ☐ Bible Study

___ **Vegetable** _____ ☐ Scripture Reading

___ **Fruit** ________ ☐ Memory Verse

___ **Milk** ________ ☐ Encouragement

___ **Fat** ________ Water ________

Exercise

Aerobic ____________

____

Strength ____________

Flexibility ____________

DAY 6: Date ____________

Morning ____________

____

____

Midday ____________

____

____

Evening ____________

____

____

Snacks ____________

____

____

___ **Meat** ________ ☐ Prayer

___ **Bread** ________ ☐ Bible Study

___ **Vegetable** _____ ☐ Scripture Reading

___ **Fruit** ________ ☐ Memory Verse

___ **Milk** ________ ☐ Encouragement

___ **Fat** ________ Water ________

Exercise

Aerobic ____________

____

Strength ____________

Flexibility ____________

DAY 7: Date ____________

Morning ____________

____

____

Midday ____________

____

____

Evening ____________

____

____

Snacks ____________

____

____

___ **Meat** ________ ☐ Prayer

___ **Bread** ________ ☐ Bible Study

___ **Vegetable** _____ ☐ Scripture Reading

___ **Fruit** ________ ☐ Memory Verse

___ **Milk** ________ ☐ Encouragement

___ **Fat** ________ Water ________

Exercise

Aerobic ____________

____

Strength ____________

Flexibility ____________

FIRST PLACE CR

Name ____________

Date ________ through ________

Week # _____ **Calorie Level** ________

Daily Exchange Plan

Level	Meat	Bread	Veggie	Fruit	Milk	Fat
1200	4-5	5-6	3	2-3	2-3	3-4
1400	5-6	6-7	3-4	3-4	2-3	3-4
1500	5-6	7-8	3-4	3-4	2-3	3-4
1600	6-7	8-9	3-4	3-4	2-3	3-4
1800	6-7	10-11	3-4	3-4	2-3	4-5
2000	6-7	11-12	4-5	4-5	2-3	4-5
2200	7-8	12-13	4-5	4-5	2-3	6-7
2400	8-9	13-14	4-5	4-5	2-3	7-8
2600	9-10	14-15	5	5	2-3	7-8
2800	9-10	15-16	5	5	2-3	9

You may always choose the high range of vegetables and fruits. Limit your high range selections to only one of the following: meat, bread, milk or fat.

______Loss ______Gain ______Maintain

___ Attendance ___ Bible Study

___ Prayer ___ Scripture Reading

___ Memory Verse ___ CR

___ Encouragement ____________

___ Exercise

Aerobic ____________

____

Strength ____________

Flexibility ____________

DAY 1: Date ______

Morning ______

Midday ______

Evening ______

Snacks ______

___ **Meat** ______ ☐ Prayer
___ **Bread** ______ ☐ Bible Study
___ **Vegetable** ______ ☐ Scripture Reading
___ **Fruit** ______ ☐ Memory Verse
___ **Milk** ______ ☐ Encouragement
___ **Fat** ______ Water ______

Exercise
Aerobic ______
Strength ______
Flexibility ______

DAY 2: Date ______

Morning ______

Midday ______

Evening ______

Snacks ______

___ **Meat** ______ ☐ Prayer
___ **Bread** ______ ☐ Bible Study
___ **Vegetable** ______ ☐ Scripture Reading
___ **Fruit** ______ ☐ Memory Verse
___ **Milk** ______ ☐ Encouragement
___ **Fat** ______ Water ______

Exercise
Aerobic ______
Strength ______
Flexibility ______

DAY 3: Date ______

Morning ______

Midday ______

Evening ______

Snacks ______

___ **Meat** ______ ☐ Prayer
___ **Bread** ______ ☐ Bible Study
___ **Vegetable** ______ ☐ Scripture Reading
___ **Fruit** ______ ☐ Memory Verse
___ **Milk** ______ ☐ Encouragement
___ **Fat** ______ Water ______

Exercise
Aerobic ______
Strength ______
Flexibility ______

DAY 4: Date ______

Morning ______

Midday ______

Evening ______

Snacks ______

___ **Meat** ______ ☐ Prayer
___ **Bread** ______ ☐ Bible Study
___ **Vegetable** ______ ☐ Scripture Reading
___ **Fruit** ______ ☐ Memory Verse
___ **Milk** ______ ☐ Encouragement
___ **Fat** ______ Water ______

Exercise
Aerobic ______
Strength ______
Flexibility ______

DAY 5: Date ____________

Morning ____________

Midday ____________

Evening ____________

Snacks ____________

___ **Meat** ______ ☐ Prayer
___ **Bread** ______ ☐ Bible Study
___ **Vegetable** ______ ☐ Scripture Reading
___ **Fruit** ______ ☐ Memory Verse
___ **Milk** ______ ☐ Encouragement
___ **Fat** ______ Water ______

Exercise
Aerobic ____________

Strength ____________
Flexibility ____________

DAY 6: Date ____________

Morning ____________

Midday ____________

Evening ____________

Snacks ____________

___ **Meat** ______ ☐ Prayer
___ **Bread** ______ ☐ Bible Study
___ **Vegetable** ______ ☐ Scripture Reading
___ **Fruit** ______ ☐ Memory Verse
___ **Milk** ______ ☐ Encouragement
___ **Fat** ______ Water ______

Exercise
Aerobic ____________

Strength ____________
Flexibility ____________

DAY 7: Date ____________

Morning ____________

Midday ____________

Evening ____________

Snacks ____________

___ **Meat** ______ ☐ Prayer
___ **Bread** ______ ☐ Bible Study
___ **Vegetable** ______ ☐ Scripture Reading
___ **Fruit** ______ ☐ Memory Verse
___ **Milk** ______ ☐ Encouragement
___ **Fat** ______ Water ______

Exercise
Aerobic ____________

Strength ____________
Flexibility ____________

FIRST PLACE CR

Name ____________

Date ______ through ______

Week # ______ **Calorie Level** ______

Daily Exchange Plan

Level	Meat	Bread	Veggie	Fruit	Milk	Fat
1200	4-5	5-6	3	2-3	2-3	3-4
1400	5-6	6-7	3-4	3-4	2-3	3-4
1500	5-6	7-8	3-4	3-4	2-3	3-4
1600	6-7	8-9	3-4	3-4	2-3	3-4
1800	6-7	10-11	3-4	3-4	2-3	4-5
2000	6-7	11-12	4-5	4-5	2-3	4-5
2200	7-8	12-13	4-5	4-5	2-3	6-7
2400	8-9	13-14	4-5	4-5	2-3	7-8
2600	9-10	14-15	5	5	2-3	7-8
2800	9-10	15-16	5	5	2-3	9

You may always choose the high range of vegetables and fruits. Limit your high range selections to only one of the following: meat, bread, milk or fat.

______ Loss ______ Gain ______ Maintain

___ Attendance ___ Bible Study
___ Prayer ___ Scripture Reading
___ Memory Verse ___ CR
___ Encouragement ____________
___ Exercise

Aerobic ____________

Strength ____________
Flexibility ____________

DAY 1: Date ______

Morning ______

______

______

Midday ______

______

______

Evening ______

______

______

Snacks ______

______

______

___ **Meat** ______ ☐ Prayer
___ **Bread** ______ ☐ Bible Study
___ **Vegetable** ______ ☐ Scripture Reading
___ **Fruit** ______ ☐ Memory Verse
___ **Milk** ______ ☐ Encouragement
___ **Fat** ______ Water ______

Exercise
Aerobic ______

______

Strength ______
Flexibility ______

DAY 2: Date ______

Morning ______

______

______

Midday ______

______

______

Evening ______

______

______

Snacks ______

______

______

___ **Meat** ______ ☐ Prayer
___ **Bread** ______ ☐ Bible Study
___ **Vegetable** ______ ☐ Scripture Reading
___ **Fruit** ______ ☐ Memory Verse
___ **Milk** ______ ☐ Encouragement
___ **Fat** ______ Water ______

Exercise
Aerobic ______

______

Strength ______
Flexibility ______

DAY 3: Date ______

Morning ______

______

______

Midday ______

______

______

Evening ______

______

______

Snacks ______

______

______

___ **Meat** ______ ☐ Prayer
___ **Bread** ______ ☐ Bible Study
___ **Vegetable** ______ ☐ Scripture Reading
___ **Fruit** ______ ☐ Memory Verse
___ **Milk** ______ ☐ Encouragement
___ **Fat** ______ Water ______

Exercise
Aerobic ______

______

Strength ______
Flexibility ______

DAY 4: Date ______

Morning ______

______

______

Midday ______

______

______

Evening ______

______

______

Snacks ______

______

______

___ **Meat** ______ ☐ Prayer
___ **Bread** ______ ☐ Bible Study
___ **Vegetable** ______ ☐ Scripture Reading
___ **Fruit** ______ ☐ Memory Verse
___ **Milk** ______ ☐ Encouragement
___ **Fat** ______ Water ______

Exercise
Aerobic ______

______

Strength ______
Flexibility ______

DAY 5: Date ____________

Morning ____________

____

____

Midday ____________

____

____

Evening ____________

____

____

Snacks ____________

____

____

___ **Meat** ________ ☐ Prayer

___ **Bread** ________ ☐ Bible Study

___ **Vegetable** ____ ☐ Scripture Reading

___ **Fruit** ________ ☐ Memory Verse

___ **Milk** ________ ☐ Encouragement

___ **Fat** ________ Water ________

Exercise

Aerobic ____________

____

Strength ____________

Flexibility ____________

DAY 6: Date ____________

Morning ____________

____

____

Midday ____________

____

____

Evening ____________

____

____

Snacks ____________

____

____

___ **Meat** ________ ☐ Prayer

___ **Bread** ________ ☐ Bible Study

___ **Vegetable** ____ ☐ Scripture Reading

___ **Fruit** ________ ☐ Memory Verse

___ **Milk** ________ ☐ Encouragement

___ **Fat** ________ Water ________

Exercise

Aerobic ____________

____

Strength ____________

Flexibility ____________

DAY 7: Date ____________

Morning ____________

____

____

Midday ____________

____

____

Evening ____________

____

____

Snacks ____________

____

____

___ **Meat** ________ ☐ Prayer

___ **Bread** ________ ☐ Bible Study

___ **Vegetable** ____ ☐ Scripture Reading

___ **Fruit** ________ ☐ Memory Verse

___ **Milk** ________ ☐ Encouragement

___ **Fat** ________ Water ________

Exercise

Aerobic ____________

____

Strength ____________

Flexibility ____________

FIRST PLACE CR

Name ____________

Date ________ through ________

Week # ______ **Calorie Level** ________

Daily Exchange Plan

Level	Meat	Bread	Veggie	Fruit	Milk	Fat
1200	4-5	5-6	3	2-3	2-3	3-4
1400	5-6	6-7	3-4	3-4	2-3	3-4
1500	5-6	7-8	3-4	3-4	2-3	3-4
1600	6-7	8-9	3-4	3-4	2-3	3-4
1800	6-7	10-11	3-4	3-4	2-3	4-5
2000	6-7	11-12	4-5	4-5	2-3	4-5
2200	7-8	12-13	4-5	4-5	2-3	6-7
2400	8-9	13-14	4-5	4-5	2-3	7-8
2600	9-10	14-15	5	5	2-3	7-8
2800	9-10	15-16	5	5	2-3	9

You may always choose the high range of vegetables and fruits. Limit your high range selections to only one of the following: meat, bread, milk or fat.

______Loss ______Gain ______Maintain

___ Attendance ___ Bible Study

___ Prayer ___ Scripture Reading

___ Memory Verse ___ CR

___ Encouragement ____________

___ Exercise

Aerobic ____________

____

Strength ____________

Flexibility ____________

DAY 1: Date ____________

Morning ____________

____

____

Midday ____________

____

____

Evening ____________

____

____

Snacks ____________

____

____

___ **Meat** ______ ☐ Prayer

___ **Bread** ______ ☐ Bible Study

___ **Vegetable** ___ ☐ Scripture Reading

___ **Fruit** ______ ☐ Memory Verse

___ **Milk** ______ ☐ Encouragement

___ **Fat** ______ Water ______

Exercise

Aerobic ____________

____

Strength ____________

Flexibility ____________

DAY 2: Date ____________

Morning ____________

____

____

Midday ____________

____

____

Evening ____________

____

____

Snacks ____________

____

____

___ **Meat** ______ ☐ Prayer

___ **Bread** ______ ☐ Bible Study

___ **Vegetable** ___ ☐ Scripture Reading

___ **Fruit** ______ ☐ Memory Verse

___ **Milk** ______ ☐ Encouragement

___ **Fat** ______ Water ______

Exercise

Aerobic ____________

____

Strength ____________

Flexibility ____________

DAY 3: Date ____________

Morning ____________

____

____

Midday ____________

____

____

Evening ____________

____

____

Snacks ____________

____

____

___ **Meat** ______ ☐ Prayer

___ **Bread** ______ ☐ Bible Study

___ **Vegetable** ___ ☐ Scripture Reading

___ **Fruit** ______ ☐ Memory Verse

___ **Milk** ______ ☐ Encouragement

___ **Fat** ______ Water ______

Exercise

Aerobic ____________

____

Strength ____________

Flexibility ____________

DAY 4: Date ____________

Morning ____________

____

____

Midday ____________

____

____

Evening ____________

____

____

Snacks ____________

____

____

___ **Meat** ______ ☐ Prayer

___ **Bread** ______ ☐ Bible Study

___ **Vegetable** ___ ☐ Scripture Reading

___ **Fruit** ______ ☐ Memory Verse

___ **Milk** ______ ☐ Encouragement

___ **Fat** ______ Water ______

Exercise

Aerobic ____________

____

Strength ____________

Flexibility ____________

DAY 5: Date ______

Morning ______

Midday ______

Evening ______

Snacks ______

___ Meat ______ ☐ Prayer
___ Bread ______ ☐ Bible Study
___ Vegetable ______ ☐ Scripture Reading
___ Fruit ______ ☐ Memory Verse
___ Milk ______ ☐ Encouragement
___ Fat ______ Water ______

Exercise
Aerobic ______

Strength ______
Flexibility ______

DAY 6: Date ______

Morning ______

Midday ______

Evening ______

Snacks ______

___ Meat ______ ☐ Prayer
___ Bread ______ ☐ Bible Study
___ Vegetable ______ ☐ Scripture Reading
___ Fruit ______ ☐ Memory Verse
___ Milk ______ ☐ Encouragement
___ Fat ______ Water ______

Exercise
Aerobic ______

Strength ______
Flexibility ______

DAY 7: Date ______

Morning ______

Midday ______

Evening ______

Snacks ______

___ Meat ______ ☐ Prayer
___ Bread ______ ☐ Bible Study
___ Vegetable ______ ☐ Scripture Reading
___ Fruit ______ ☐ Memory Verse
___ Milk ______ ☐ Encouragement
___ Fat ______ Water ______

Exercise
Aerobic ______

Strength ______
Flexibility ______

FIRST PLACE CR

Name ______
Date ______ through ______
Week # ______ Calorie Level ______

Daily Exchange Plan

Level	Meat	Bread	Veggie	Fruit	Milk	Fat
1200	4-5	5-6	3	2-3	2-3	3-4
1400	5-6	6-7	3-4	3-4	2-3	3-4
1500	5-6	7-8	3-4	3-4	2-3	3-4
1600	6-7	8-9	3-4	3-4	2-3	3-4
1800	6-7	10-11	3-4	3-4	2-3	4-5
2000	6-7	11-12	4-5	4-5	2-3	4-5
2200	7-8	12-13	4-5	4-5	2-3	6-7
2400	8-9	13-14	4-5	4-5	2-3	7-8
2600	9-10	14-15	5	5	2-3	7-8
2800	9-10	15-16	5	5	2-3	9

You may always choose the high range of vegetables and fruits. Limit your high range selections to only one of the following: meat, bread, milk or fat.

______ Loss ______ Gain ______ Maintain

___ Attendance ___ Bible Study
___ Prayer ___ Scripture Reading
___ Memory Verse ___ CR
___ Encouragement ______
___ Exercise
Aerobic ______

Strength ______
Flexibility ______

DAY 1: Date ____________

Morning ____________

____

____

Midday ____________

____

____

Evening ____________

____

____

Snacks ____________

____

____

___ **Meat** ________ ☐ Prayer

___ **Bread** ________ ☐ Bible Study

___ **Vegetable** ________ ☐ Scripture Reading

___ **Fruit** ________ ☐ Memory Verse

___ **Milk** ________ ☐ Encouragement

___ **Fat** ________ Water ________

Exercise

Aerobic ____________

____

Strength ____________

Flexibility ____________

DAY 2: Date ____________

Morning ____________

____

____

Midday ____________

____

____

Evening ____________

____

____

Snacks ____________

____

____

___ **Meat** ________ ☐ Prayer

___ **Bread** ________ ☐ Bible Study

___ **Vegetable** ________ ☐ Scripture Reading

___ **Fruit** ________ ☐ Memory Verse

___ **Milk** ________ ☐ Encouragement

___ **Fat** ________ Water ________

Exercise

Aerobic ____________

____

Strength ____________

Flexibility ____________

DAY 3: Date ____________

Morning ____________

____

____

Midday ____________

____

____

Evening ____________

____

____

Snacks ____________

____

____

___ **Meat** ________ ☐ Prayer

___ **Bread** ________ ☐ Bible Study

___ **Vegetable** ________ ☐ Scripture Reading

___ **Fruit** ________ ☐ Memory Verse

___ **Milk** ________ ☐ Encouragement

___ **Fat** ________ Water ________

Exercise

Aerobic ____________

____

Strength ____________

Flexibility ____________

DAY 4: Date ____________

Morning ____________

____

____

Midday ____________

____

____

Evening ____________

____

____

Snacks ____________

____

____

___ **Meat** ________ ☐ Prayer

___ **Bread** ________ ☐ Bible Study

___ **Vegetable** ________ ☐ Scripture Reading

___ **Fruit** ________ ☐ Memory Verse

___ **Milk** ________ ☐ Encouragement

___ **Fat** ________ Water ________

Exercise

Aerobic ____________

____

Strength ____________

Flexibility ____________

DAY 5: Date ____________

Morning ____________

____

____

Midday ____________

____

____

Evening ____________

____

____

Snacks ____________

____

____

___ **Meat** ______ ☐ Prayer

___ **Bread** ______ ☐ Bible Study

___ **Vegetable** ______ ☐ Scripture Reading

___ **Fruit** ______ ☐ Memory Verse

___ **Milk** ______ ☐ Encouragement

___ **Fat** ______ Water ______

Exercise

Aerobic ____________

____

Strength ____________

Flexibility ____________

DAY 6: Date ____________

Morning ____________

____

____

Midday ____________

____

____

Evening ____________

____

____

Snacks ____________

____

____

___ **Meat** ______ ☐ Prayer

___ **Bread** ______ ☐ Bible Study

___ **Vegetable** ______ ☐ Scripture Reading

___ **Fruit** ______ ☐ Memory Verse

___ **Milk** ______ ☐ Encouragement

___ **Fat** ______ Water ______

Exercise

Aerobic ____________

____

Strength ____________

Flexibility ____________

DAY 7: Date ____________

Morning ____________

____

____

Midday ____________

____

____

Evening ____________

____

____

Snacks ____________

____

____

___ **Meat** ______ ☐ Prayer

___ **Bread** ______ ☐ Bible Study

___ **Vegetable** ______ ☐ Scripture Reading

___ **Fruit** ______ ☐ Memory Verse

___ **Milk** ______ ☐ Encouragement

___ **Fat** ______ Water ______

Exercise

Aerobic ____________

____

Strength ____________

Flexibility ____________

FIRST PLACE CR

Name ____________

Date ______ through ______

Week # ______ **Calorie Level** ______

Daily Exchange Plan

Level	Meat	Bread	Veggie	Fruit	Milk	Fat
1200	4-5	5-6	3	2-3	2-3	3-4
1400	5-6	6-7	3-4	3-4	2-3	3-4
1500	5-6	7-8	3-4	3-4	2-3	3-4
1600	6-7	8-9	3-4	3-4	2-3	3-4
1800	6-7	10-11	3-4	3-4	2-3	4-5
2000	6-7	11-12	4-5	4-5	2-3	4-5
2200	7-8	12-13	4-5	4-5	2-3	6-7
2400	8-9	13-14	4-5	4-5	2-3	7-8
2600	9-10	14-15	5	5	2-3	7-8
2800	9-10	15-16	5	5	2-3	9

You may always choose the high range of vegetables and fruits. Limit your high range selections to only one of the following: meat, bread, milk or fat.

______ Loss ______ Gain ______ Maintain

___ Attendance ___ Bible Study

___ Prayer ___ Scripture Reading

___ Memory Verse ___ CR

___ Encouragement ____________

___ Exercise

Aerobic ____________

____

Strength ____________

Flexibility ____________

DAY 1: Date ____________

Morning ____________

Midday ____________

Evening ____________

Snacks ____________

___ **Meat** ________ ☐ Prayer
___ **Bread** ________ ☐ Bible Study
___ **Vegetable** ____ ☐ Scripture Reading
___ **Fruit** ________ ☐ Memory Verse
___ **Milk** ________ ☐ Encouragement
___ **Fat** ________ Water ________

Exercise
Aerobic ____________
Strength ____________
Flexibility ____________

DAY 2: Date ____________

Morning ____________

Midday ____________

Evening ____________

Snacks ____________

___ **Meat** ________ ☐ Prayer
___ **Bread** ________ ☐ Bible Study
___ **Vegetable** ____ ☐ Scripture Reading
___ **Fruit** ________ ☐ Memory Verse
___ **Milk** ________ ☐ Encouragement
___ **Fat** ________ Water ________

Exercise
Aerobic ____________
Strength ____________
Flexibility ____________

DAY 3: Date ____________

Morning ____________

Midday ____________

Evening ____________

Snacks ____________

___ **Meat** ________ ☐ Prayer
___ **Bread** ________ ☐ Bible Study
___ **Vegetable** ____ ☐ Scripture Reading
___ **Fruit** ________ ☐ Memory Verse
___ **Milk** ________ ☐ Encouragement
___ **Fat** ________ Water ________

Exercise
Aerobic ____________
Strength ____________
Flexibility ____________

DAY 4: Date ____________

Morning ____________

Midday ____________

Evening ____________

Snacks ____________

___ **Meat** ________ ☐ Prayer
___ **Bread** ________ ☐ Bible Study
___ **Vegetable** ____ ☐ Scripture Reading
___ **Fruit** ________ ☐ Memory Verse
___ **Milk** ________ ☐ Encouragement
___ **Fat** ________ Water ________

Exercise
Aerobic ____________
Strength ____________
Flexibility ____________

DAY 5: Date ____________

Morning ____________

Midday ____________

Evening ____________

Snacks ____________

___ Meat ______ ☐ Prayer
___ Bread ______ ☐ Bible Study
___ Vegetable ______ ☐ Scripture Reading
___ Fruit ______ ☐ Memory Verse
___ Milk ______ ☐ Encouragement
___ Fat ______ Water ______

Exercise
Aerobic ____________

Strength ____________
Flexibility ____________

DAY 6: Date ____________

Morning ____________

Midday ____________

Evening ____________

Snacks ____________

___ Meat ______ ☐ Prayer
___ Bread ______ ☐ Bible Study
___ Vegetable ______ ☐ Scripture Reading
___ Fruit ______ ☐ Memory Verse
___ Milk ______ ☐ Encouragement
___ Fat ______ Water ______

Exercise
Aerobic ____________

Strength ____________
Flexibility ____________

DAY 7: Date ____________

Morning ____________

Midday ____________

Evening ____________

Snacks ____________

___ Meat ______ ☐ Prayer
___ Bread ______ ☐ Bible Study
___ Vegetable ______ ☐ Scripture Reading
___ Fruit ______ ☐ Memory Verse
___ Milk ______ ☐ Encouragement
___ Fat ______ Water ______

Exercise
Aerobic ____________

Strength ____________
Flexibility ____________

FIRST PLACE CR

Name ____________
Date ______ through ______
Week # ______ Calorie Level ______

Daily Exchange Plan

Level	Meat	Bread	Veggie	Fruit	Milk	Fat
1200	4-5	5-6	3	2-3	2-3	3-4
1400	5-6	6-7	3-4	3-4	2-3	3-4
1500	5-6	7-8	3-4	3-4	2-3	3-4
1600	6-7	8-9	3-4	3-4	2-3	3-4
1800	6-7	10-11	3-4	3-4	2-3	4-5
2000	6-7	11-12	4-5	4-5	2-3	4-5
2200	7-8	12-13	4-5	4-5	2-3	6-7
2400	8-9	13-14	4-5	4-5	2-3	7-8
2600	9-10	14-15	5	5	2-3	7-8
2800	9-10	15-16	5	5	2-3	9

You may always choose the high range of vegetables and fruits. Limit your high range selections to only one of the following: meat, bread, milk or fat.

______ Loss ______ Gain ______ Maintain

___ Attendance ___ Bible Study
___ Prayer ___ Scripture Reading
___ Memory Verse ___ CR
___ Encouragement ____________
___ Exercise
Aerobic ____________

Strength ____________
Flexibility ____________

DAY 1: Date ____________

Morning ____________

Midday ____________

Evening ____________

Snacks ____________

___ **Meat** ______ ☐ Prayer
___ **Bread** ______ ☐ Bible Study
___ **Vegetable** ______ ☐ Scripture Reading
___ **Fruit** ______ ☐ Memory Verse
___ **Milk** ______ ☐ Encouragement
___ **Fat** ______ Water ______

Exercise
Aerobic ____________
Strength ____________
Flexibility ____________

DAY 2: Date ____________

Morning ____________

Midday ____________

Evening ____________

Snacks ____________

___ **Meat** ______ ☐ Prayer
___ **Bread** ______ ☐ Bible Study
___ **Vegetable** ______ ☐ Scripture Reading
___ **Fruit** ______ ☐ Memory Verse
___ **Milk** ______ ☐ Encouragement
___ **Fat** ______ Water ______

Exercise
Aerobic ____________
Strength ____________
Flexibility ____________

DAY 3: Date ____________

Morning ____________

Midday ____________

Evening ____________

Snacks ____________

___ **Meat** ______ ☐ Prayer
___ **Bread** ______ ☐ Bible Study
___ **Vegetable** ______ ☐ Scripture Reading
___ **Fruit** ______ ☐ Memory Verse
___ **Milk** ______ ☐ Encouragement
___ **Fat** ______ Water ______

Exercise
Aerobic ____________
Strength ____________
Flexibility ____________

DAY 4: Date ____________

Morning ____________

Midday ____________

Evening ____________

Snacks ____________

___ **Meat** ______ ☐ Prayer
___ **Bread** ______ ☐ Bible Study
___ **Vegetable** ______ ☐ Scripture Reading
___ **Fruit** ______ ☐ Memory Verse
___ **Milk** ______ ☐ Encouragement
___ **Fat** ______ Water ______

Exercise
Aerobic ____________
Strength ____________
Flexibility ____________

DAY 5: Date ______

Morning ______

Midday ______

Evening ______

Snacks ______

___ Meat ______ ☐ Prayer
___ Bread ______ ☐ Bible Study
___ Vegetable ______ ☐ Scripture Reading
___ Fruit ______ ☐ Memory Verse
___ Milk ______ ☐ Encouragement
___ Fat ______ Water ______

Exercise
Aerobic ______
Strength ______
Flexibility ______

DAY 6: Date ______

Morning ______

Midday ______

Evening ______

Snacks ______

___ Meat ______ ☐ Prayer
___ Bread ______ ☐ Bible Study
___ Vegetable ______ ☐ Scripture Reading
___ Fruit ______ ☐ Memory Verse
___ Milk ______ ☐ Encouragement
___ Fat ______ Water ______

Exercise
Aerobic ______
Strength ______
Flexibility ______

DAY 7: Date ______

Morning ______

Midday ______

Evening ______

Snacks ______

___ Meat ______ ☐ Prayer
___ Bread ______ ☐ Bible Study
___ Vegetable ______ ☐ Scripture Reading
___ Fruit ______ ☐ Memory Verse
___ Milk ______ ☐ Encouragement
___ Fat ______ Water ______

Exercise
Aerobic ______
Strength ______
Flexibility ______

FIRST PLACE CR

Name ______
Date ______ through ______
Week # ______ Calorie Level ______

Daily Exchange Plan

Level	Meat	Bread	Veggie	Fruit	Milk	Fat
1200	4-5	5-6	3	2-3	2-3	3-4
1400	5-6	6-7	3-4	3-4	2-3	3-4
1500	5-6	7-8	3-4	3-4	2-3	3-4
1600	6-7	8-9	3-4	3-4	2-3	3-4
1800	6-7	10-11	3-4	3-4	2-3	4-5
2000	6-7	11-12	4-5	4-5	2-3	4-5
2200	7-8	12-13	4-5	4-5	2-3	6-7
2400	8-9	13-14	4-5	4-5	2-3	7-8
2600	9-10	14-15	5	5	2-3	7-8
2800	9-10	15-16	5	5	2-3	9

You may always choose the high range of vegetables and fruits. Limit your high range selections to only one of the following: meat, bread, milk or fat.

______ Loss ______ Gain ______ Maintain

___ Attendance ___ Bible Study
___ Prayer ___ Scripture Reading
___ Memory Verse ___ CR
___ Encouragement ______
___ Exercise
Aerobic ______
Strength ______
Flexibility ______

DAY 1: Date ____________

Morning ____________

Midday ____________

Evening ____________

Snacks ____________

___ Meat ______ ☐ Prayer
___ Bread ______ ☐ Bible Study
___ Vegetable ___ ☐ Scripture Reading
___ Fruit ______ ☐ Memory Verse
___ Milk ______ ☐ Encouragement
___ Fat ______ Water ______

Exercise
Aerobic ____________
Strength ____________
Flexibility ____________

DAY 2: Date ____________

Morning ____________

Midday ____________

Evening ____________

Snacks ____________

___ Meat ______ ☐ Prayer
___ Bread ______ ☐ Bible Study
___ Vegetable ___ ☐ Scripture Reading
___ Fruit ______ ☐ Memory Verse
___ Milk ______ ☐ Encouragement
___ Fat ______ Water ______

Exercise
Aerobic ____________
Strength ____________
Flexibility ____________

DAY 3: Date ____________

Morning ____________

Midday ____________

Evening ____________

Snacks ____________

___ Meat ______ ☐ Prayer
___ Bread ______ ☐ Bible Study
___ Vegetable ___ ☐ Scripture Reading
___ Fruit ______ ☐ Memory Verse
___ Milk ______ ☐ Encouragement
___ Fat ______ Water ______

Exercise
Aerobic ____________
Strength ____________
Flexibility ____________

DAY 4: Date ____________

Morning ____________

Midday ____________

Evening ____________

Snacks ____________

___ Meat ______ ☐ Prayer
___ Bread ______ ☐ Bible Study
___ Vegetable ___ ☐ Scripture Reading
___ Fruit ______ ☐ Memory Verse
___ Milk ______ ☐ Encouragement
___ Fat ______ Water ______

Exercise
Aerobic ____________
Strength ____________
Flexibility ____________

DAY 5: Date ________

Morning ________

____

____

Midday ________

____

____

Evening ________

____

____

Snacks ________

____

____

___ **Meat** ______ ☐ Prayer

___ **Bread** ______ ☐ Bible Study

___ **Vegetable** ______ ☐ Scripture Reading

___ **Fruit** ______ ☐ Memory Verse

___ **Milk** ______ ☐ Encouragement

___ **Fat** ______ Water ______

Exercise

Aerobic ________

____

Strength ________

Flexibility ________

DAY 6: Date ________

Morning ________

____

____

Midday ________

____

____

Evening ________

____

____

Snacks ________

____

____

___ **Meat** ______ ☐ Prayer

___ **Bread** ______ ☐ Bible Study

___ **Vegetable** ______ ☐ Scripture Reading

___ **Fruit** ______ ☐ Memory Verse

___ **Milk** ______ ☐ Encouragement

___ **Fat** ______ Water ______

Exercise

Aerobic ________

____

Strength ________

Flexibility ________

DAY 7: Date ________

Morning ________

____

____

Midday ________

____

____

Evening ________

____

____

Snacks ________

____

____

___ **Meat** ______ ☐ Prayer

___ **Bread** ______ ☐ Bible Study

___ **Vegetable** ______ ☐ Scripture Reading

___ **Fruit** ______ ☐ Memory Verse

___ **Milk** ______ ☐ Encouragement

___ **Fat** ______ Water ______

Exercise

Aerobic ________

____

Strength ________

Flexibility ________

FIRST PLACE CR

Name ________

Date ______ through ______

Week # ______ **Calorie Level** ______

Daily Exchange Plan

Level	Meat	Bread	Veggie	Fruit	Milk	Fat
1200	4-5	5-6	3	2-3	2-3	3-4
1400	5-6	6-7	3-4	3-4	2-3	3-4
1500	5-6	7-8	3-4	3-4	2-3	3-4
1600	6-7	8-9	3-4	3-4	2-3	3-4
1800	6-7	10-11	3-4	3-4	2-3	4-5
2000	6-7	11-12	4-5	4-5	2-3	4-5
2200	7-8	12-13	4-5	4-5	2-3	6-7
2400	8-9	13-14	4-5	4-5	2-3	7-8
2600	9-10	14-15	5	5	2-3	7-8
2800	9-10	15-16	5	5	2-3	9

You may always choose the high range of vegetables and fruits. Limit your high range selections to only one of the following: meat, bread, milk or fat.

______ Loss ______ Gain ______ Maintain

___ Attendance ___ Bible Study

___ Prayer ___ Scripture Reading

___ Memory Verse ___ CR

___ Encouragement ________

___ Exercise

Aerobic ________

____

Strength ________

Flexibility ________

DAY 1: Date ____________

Morning ____________

____

____

Midday ____________

____

____

Evening ____________

____

____

Snacks ____________

____

____

___ **Meat** ________ ☐ Prayer

___ **Bread** ________ ☐ Bible Study

___ **Vegetable** _____ ☐ Scripture Reading

___ **Fruit** ________ ☐ Memory Verse

___ **Milk** ________ ☐ Encouragement

___ **Fat** ________ Water ________

Exercise

Aerobic ____________

____

Strength ____________

Flexibility ____________

DAY 2: Date ____________

Morning ____________

____

____

Midday ____________

____

____

Evening ____________

____

____

Snacks ____________

____

____

___ **Meat** ________ ☐ Prayer

___ **Bread** ________ ☐ Bible Study

___ **Vegetable** _____ ☐ Scripture Reading

___ **Fruit** ________ ☐ Memory Verse

___ **Milk** ________ ☐ Encouragement

___ **Fat** ________ Water ________

Exercise

Aerobic ____________

____

Strength ____________

Flexibility ____________

DAY 3: Date ____________

Morning ____________

____

____

Midday ____________

____

____

Evening ____________

____

____

Snacks ____________

____

____

___ **Meat** ________ ☐ Prayer

___ **Bread** ________ ☐ Bible Study

___ **Vegetable** _____ ☐ Scripture Reading

___ **Fruit** ________ ☐ Memory Verse

___ **Milk** ________ ☐ Encouragement

___ **Fat** ________ Water ________

Exercise

Aerobic ____________

____

Strength ____________

Flexibility ____________

DAY 4: Date ____________

Morning ____________

____

____

Midday ____________

____

____

Evening ____________

____

____

Snacks ____________

____

____

___ **Meat** ________ ☐ Prayer

___ **Bread** ________ ☐ Bible Study

___ **Vegetable** _____ ☐ Scripture Reading

___ **Fruit** ________ ☐ Memory Verse

___ **Milk** ________ ☐ Encouragement

___ **Fat** ________ Water ________

Exercise

Aerobic ____________

____

Strength ____________

Flexibility ____________

CONTRIBUTORS

Jody Wilkinson, M.D., M.S., the writer of the Wellness Worksheets for this study, is a physician and exercise physiologist at the Cooper Institute in Dallas, Texas. He trained at the University of Texas Health Science Center in San Antonio, Texas, and Baylor University Medical Center in Dallas. Dr. Wilkinson conducts research on physical activity, nutrition and weight management and has worked with the American Heart Association to develop a health program. He believes strongly in using biblical teaching to motivate people to take care of their physical bodies and enjoy abundant living. Jody and his wife, Natalie, have been married 10 years and have two daughters, Jordan and Sarah, and twin sons, Joel and Cooper.

Scott Wilson, C.E.C., A.A.C., the author of the menu plans in this study, has been cooking professionally for 23 years. A certified executive chef with the American Culinary Federation, he currently works in the Greater Atlanta area as a personal chef and food consultant. Along with serving as the national food consultant for First Place, he is a part-time nutrition teacher at Life University and chef/host of a cable cooking show in the Atlanta area, "Cooking 4 Life." Scott has also authored two cookbooks, *Dining Under the Magnolia* and *Healthy Home Cooking*. In his spare time, he is active in church work and spends time with his wife, Jennifer, and their daughter, Katie.

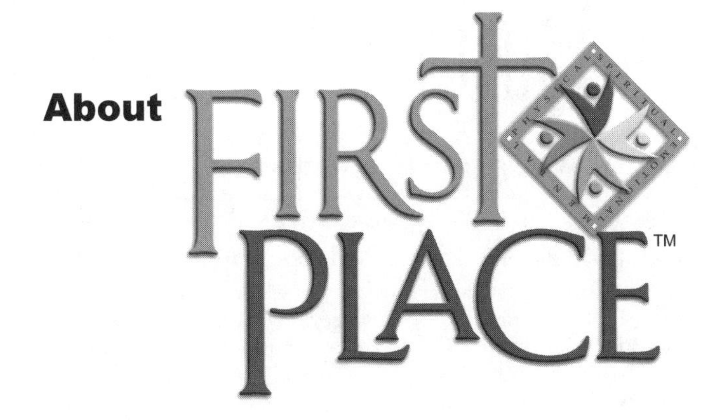

First Place was founded under the providence of God and with the conviction that there is a need for a program which will train the minds, develop the moral character and enrich the spiritual lives of all those who may come within the sphere of its influence.

First Place is dedicated to providing quality information for development of a physical, emotional and spiritual environment leading to a life that honors God in Jesus Christ. As a health-oriented program, First Place will stress the highest excellence and proficiency in instruction with a goal of developing within each participant mastery of all the basics of a lasting healthy lifestyle, so that all may achieve their highest potential in body, mind and spirit. The spiritual development of each participant shall be given high priority so that each may come to the knowledge of Jesus Christ and God's plan and purpose for each life.

First Place offers instruction, encouragement and support to help members experience a more abundant life. Please contact the First Place national office in Houston, Texas at (800) 727-5223 for information on the following resources:

- ❖ Training Opportunities
- ❖ Conferences/Rallies
- ❖ Workshops
- ❖ Fitness Weeks

Send personal testimonies to:

First Place
7401 Katy Freeway
Houston, TX 77024

Join the First Place community at **www.firstplace.org**

Bible Studies to Help You Put Christ First

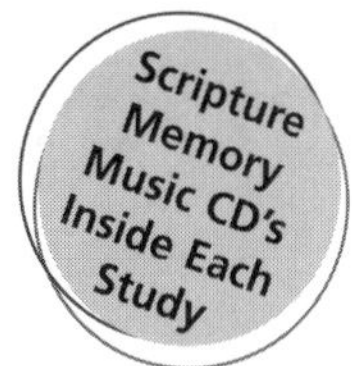

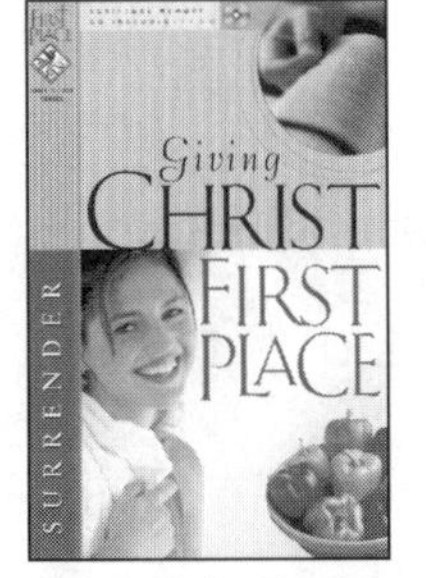

Giving Christ First Place
Bible Study
ISBN 08307.28643
Now Available

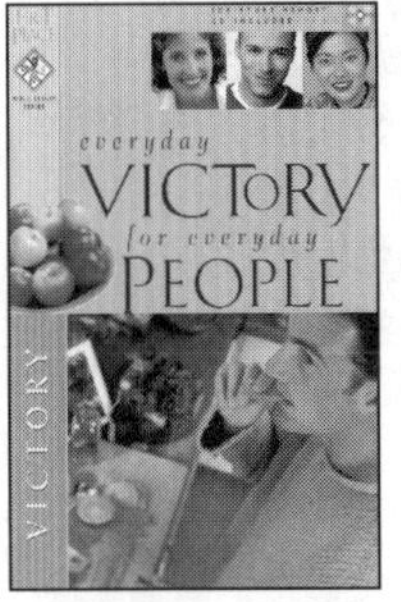

Everyday Victory for Everyday People
Bible Study
ISBN 08307.28651
Now Available

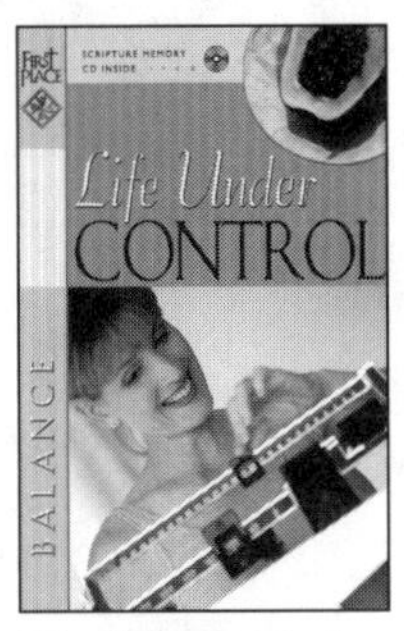

Life Under Control
Bible Study
ISBN 08307.29305
Now Available

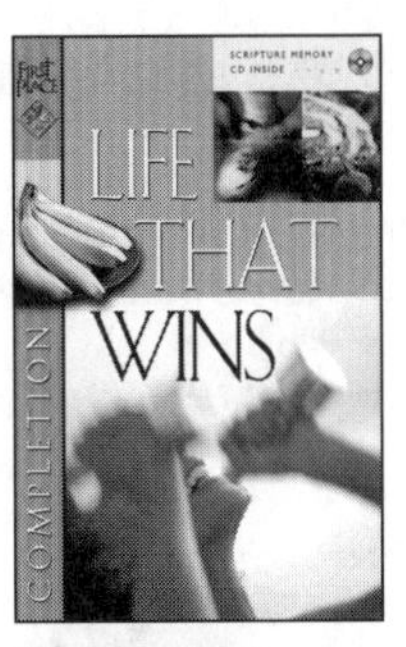

Life That Wins
Bible Study
ISBN 08307.29240
Now Available

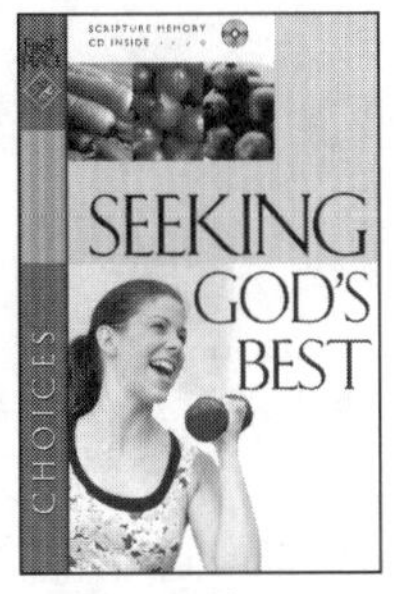

Seeking God's Best
Bible Study
ISBN 08307.29259
Available April 2002
Now Available

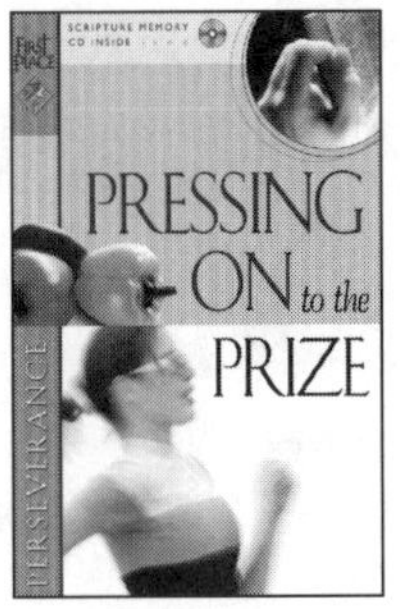

Pressing On to the Prize
Bible Study
ISBN 08307.29267
Available April 2002
Now Available

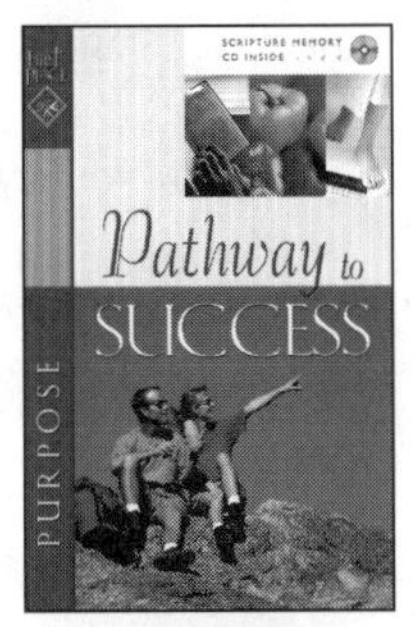

Pathway to Success
Bible Study
ISBN 08307.29275
Available July 2002

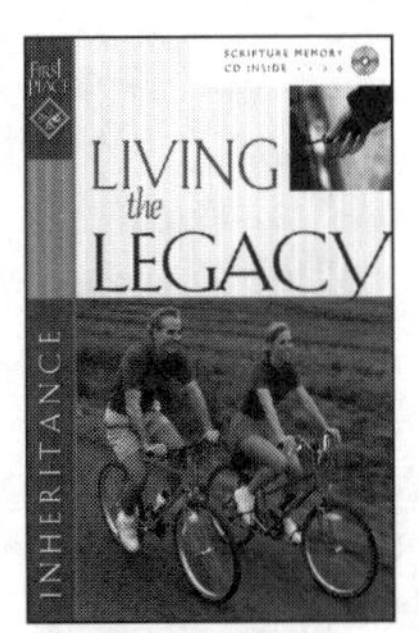

Living the Legacy
Bible Study
ISBN 08307.29283
Available July 2002

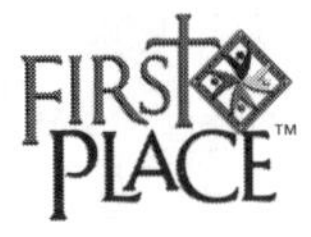

Available at your local Christian bookstore or by calling 1-800-4-GOSPEL.

Join the First Place community at **www.firstplace.org**

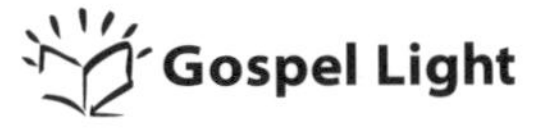

11062

Plant God's Word in Your Heart.

Walking in the Word Scripture Memory Music & More!

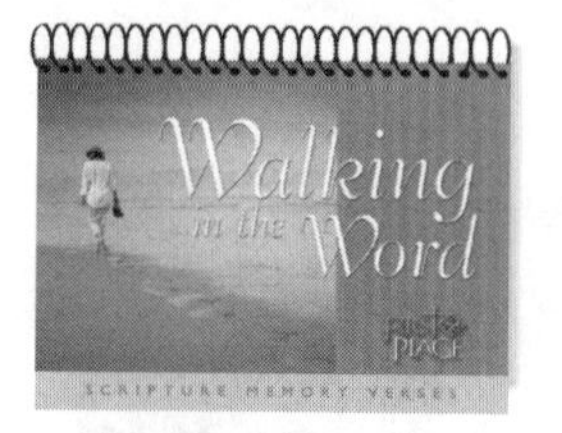

Walking in the Word Scripture Memory Verses
Easel Flip Book
ISBN 08307.28996

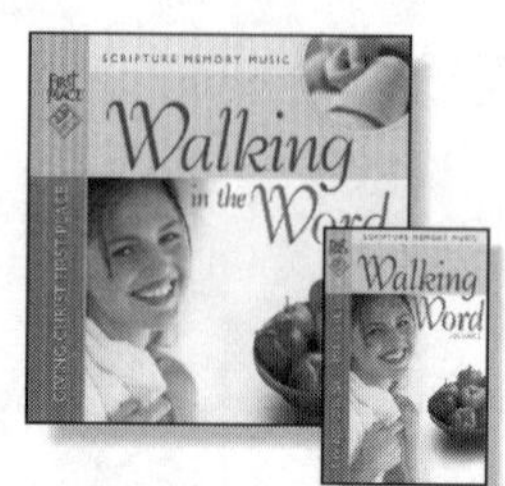

Volume 1: Giving Christ First Place
CD • UPC 607135.005902
Cassette • UPC 607135.005919

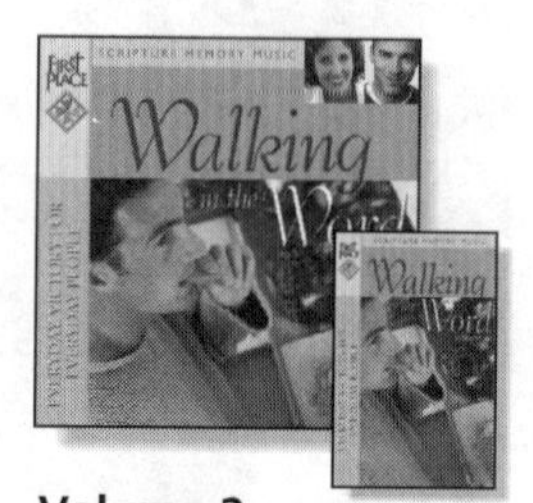

Volume 2: Everyday Victory for Everyday People
CD • UPC 607135.005926
Cassette • UPC 607135.005933

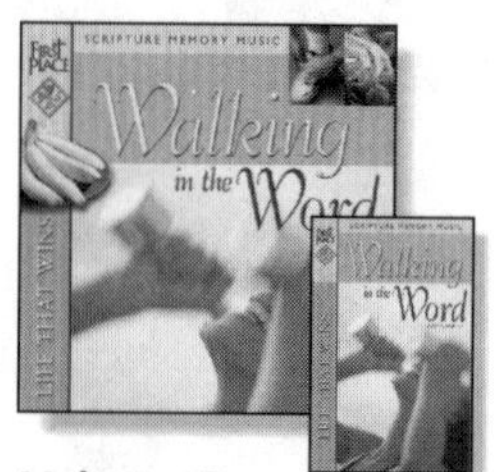

Volume 3: Life That Wins
CD • UPC 607135.006237
Cassette • UPC 607135.006220

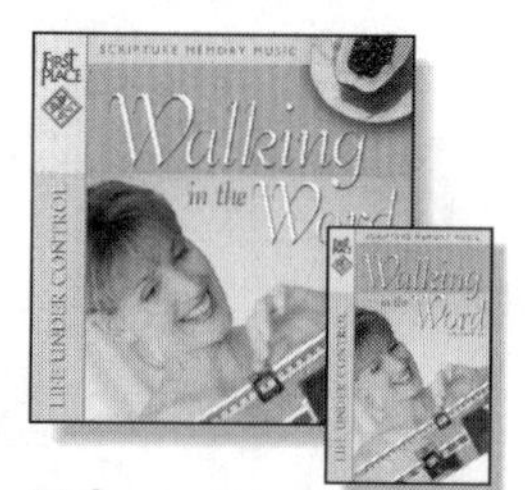

Volume 4: Life Under Control
CD • UPC 607135.006213
Cassette • UPC 607135.006206

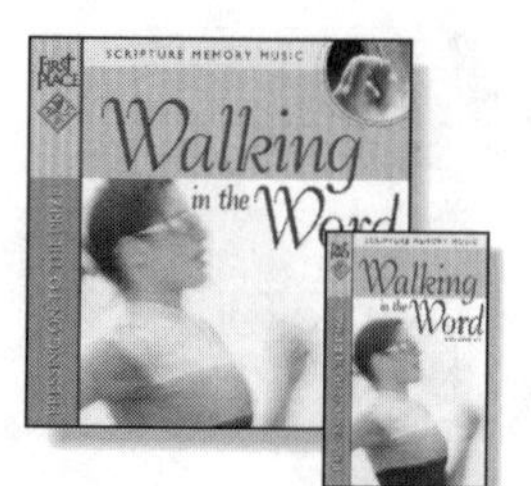

Volume 5: Pressing On to the Prize
CD • UPC 607135.006268
Cassette • UPC 607135.006275

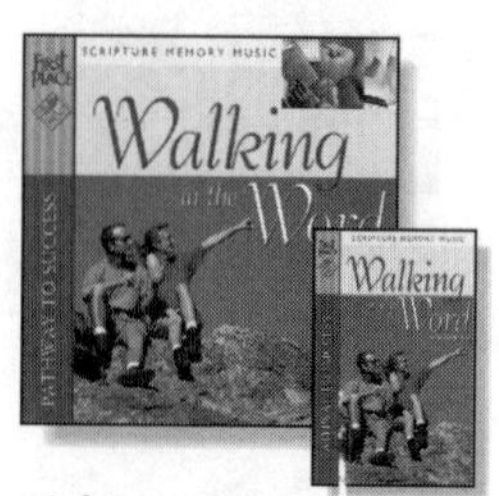

Volume 6: Pathway to Success
CD • UPC 607135.006282
Cassette • UPC 607135.006299

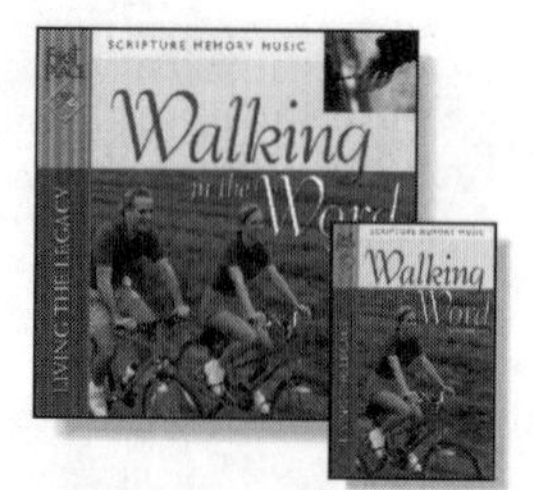

Volume 7: Living the Legacy
CD • UPC 607135.006305
Cassette • UPC 607135.006312

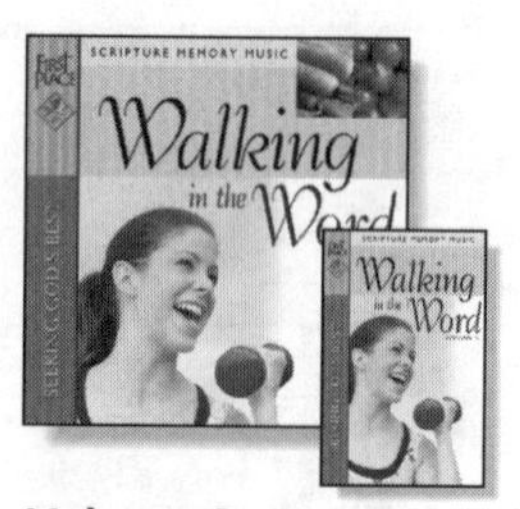

Volume 8: Seeking God's Best
CD • UPC 607135.006244
Cassette • UPC 607135.006251

Available at your local Christian bookstore
or by calling **1-800-4-GOSPEL.**

11080

Join the First Place community at **www.firstplace.org.**

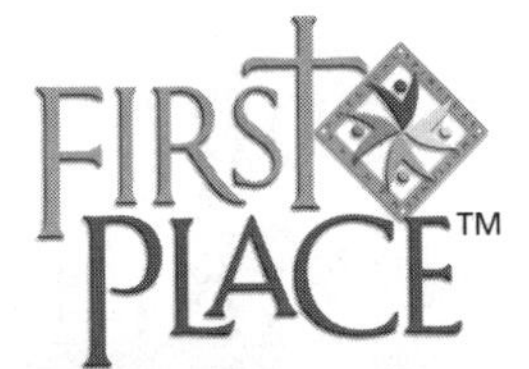

Available from your Gospel Light supplier

First Place Resource Order Form

TITLE	ISBN/SPCN	QTY	PRICE	ITEM TOTAL
First Place Group Starter Kit ($198 Value!)	08307.28708		149.99	
First Place Member's Kit ($101 Value!)	08307.28694		79.99	
First Place (Lewis/Whalin) (included in Group Starter Kit)	08307.28635		18.99	
Choosing to Change (Lewis) (included in Member's and Group Starter Kits)	08307.28627		8.99	
Giving Christ First Place Bible Study w/Scripture Memory Music CD (included in Group Starter Kit)	08307.28643		19.99	
Everyday Victory for Everyday People Bible Study w/Scripture Memory Music CD	08307.28651		19.99	
Life That Wins Bible Study w/ Scripture Memory Music CD	08307.29240		19.99	
Life Under Control Bible Study w/ Scripture Memory Music CD	08307.29305		19.99	
Pressing On to the Prize Bible Study w/ Scripture Memory Music CD	08307.29267		19.99	
Seeking God's Best Bible Study w/ Scripture Memory Music CD	08307.29259		19.99	
Living the Legacy Bible Study w/ Scripture Memory Music CD	08307.29283		19.99	
Pathway to Success Bible Study w/ Scripture Memory Music CD	08307.29275		19.99	
Prayer Journal (included in Member's Kit)	08307.29003		9.99	
Motivational Audiocassettes (pkg. of 4) (included in Member's Kit)	607135.005988		29.99	
Commitment Records (pkg. o f 13) (included in Member's Kit)	08307.29011		6.99	
Scripture Memory Verses: Walking in the Word (included in Member's Kit)	08307.28996		14.99	
Leader's Guide (included in Group Starter Kit)	08307.28678		19.99	
Food Exchange Plan Video (included in Group Starter Kit)	607135.006138		29.99	
Orientation Video (included in Group Starter Kit)	607135.005940		29.99	
Nine Commitments Video (included in Group Starter Kit)	607135.005957		39.99	
Giving Christ First Place Scripture Memory Music CD	607135.005902		9.99	
Giving Christ First Place Scripture Memory Music Cassette	607135.005919		6.99	
Everyday Victory for Everyday People Scripture Memory Music CD	607135.005926		9.99	
Everyday Victory for Everyday People Scripture Memory Music Cassette	607135.005933		6.99	
Life Under Control Scripture Memory Music CD	607135.006213		9.99	
Life Under Control Scripture Memory Music Cassette	607135.006206		6.99	
Life That Wins Scripture Memory Music CD	607135.006237		9.99	
Life That Wins Scripture Memory Music Cassette	607135.006220		6.99	
Seeking God's Best Scripture Memory Music CD	607135.006244		9.99	
Seeking God's Best Scripture Memory Music Cassette	607135.006251		6.99	
Pressing On to the Prize Scripture Memory Music CD	607135.006268		9.99	
Pressing On to the Prize Scripture Memory Music Cassette	607135.006275		6.99	
Pathway to Success Scripture Memory Music CD	607135.006282		9.99	
Pathway to Success Scripture Memory Music Cassette	607135.006299		6.99	
Living the Legacy Scripture Memory Music CD	607135.006305		9.99	
Living the Legacy Scripture Memory Music Cassette	607135.006312		6.99	

PRICES SUBJECT TO CHANGE.

Total : $________

11052